MW00684974

Brain Imaging in Affective Disorders

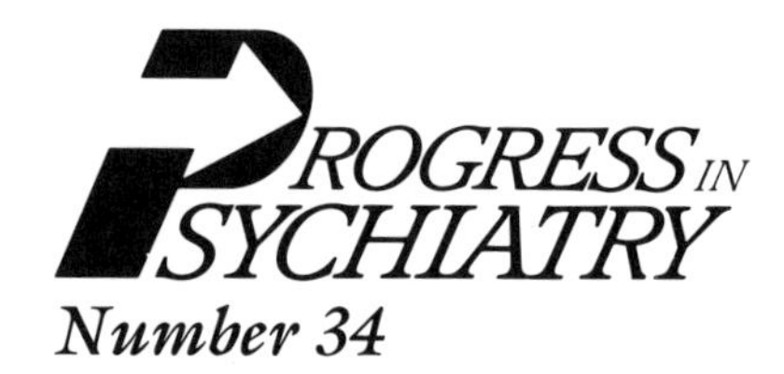

Number 34

David Spiegel, M.D.
Series Editor

Brain Imaging in Affective Disorders

Edited by
Peter Hauser, M.D.

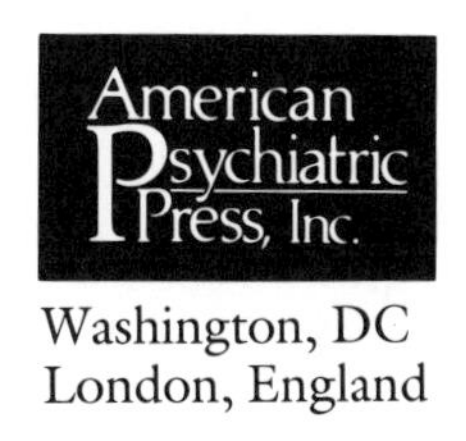

Washington, DC
London, England

Note: The authors have worked to ensure that all information in this book concerning drug dosages, schedules, and routes of administration is accurate as of the time of publication and consistent with standards set by the U.S. Food and Drug Administration and the general medical community. As medical research and practice advance, however, therapeutic standards may change. For this reason and because human and mechanical errors sometimes occur, we recommend that readers follow the advice of a physician who is directly involved in their care or the care of a member of their family.

Manufactured in the United States of America on acid-free paper.

First Edition 94 93 92 91 4 3 2 1

American Psychiatric Press, Inc.
1400 K Street, N.W., Washington, DC, 20005

Library of Congress Cataloging-in-Publication Data

Brain imaging in affective disorders/edited by Peter Hauser.—1st ed.
p. cm. — (Progress in psychiatry series: no. 34)
Includes bibliographical references.
ISBN 0-88048-456-X (alk. paper)
1. Affective disorders—Imaging. 2. Brain—Imaging. 3. Affective disorders—Diagnosis. I. Hauser, Peter, 1955– II. Series: Progress in psychiatry series ; 34.
[DNLM: 1. Affective Disorders—diagnosis. 2. Affective Disorders—pathology. 3. Brain—pathology. 4. Diagnostic Imaging—methods. WM 207 B814]
RC537.B673 1991
616.85'270757—dc20
DNLM/DLC
for Library of Congress 91-4539
CIP

British Library Cataloguing in Publication Data

A CIP record is available from the British Library.

Contents

Contributors

Lewis R. Baxter, Jr., M.D.
Department of Psychiatry and Biobehavioral Sciences, The Neuropsychiatric Institute, University of California, Los Angeles, Los Angeles, California

Joseph B. Bryer, M.D.
Department of Psychiatry and Behavioral Sciences, Johns Hopkins School of Medicine, Baltimore, Maryland

C. Edward Coffey, M.D.
Allegheny Neuropsychiatric Institute, Oakdale, Pennsylvania

Renee M. Dupont, M.D.
Department of Psychiatry, University of California, San Diego, and San Diego Veterans Administration Medical Center, La Jolla, California

Barry H. Guze, M.D.
Department of Psychiatry and Biobehavioral Sciences, The Neuropsychiatric Institute, University of California, Los Angeles, Los Angeles, California

Peter Hauser, M.D.
National Institute of Diabetes, Digestive, and Kidney Diseases (previously at the National Institute of Mental Health), National Institutes of Health, Bethesda, Maryland

Dilip Jeste, M.D.
Department of Psychiatry, University of California, San Diego, and San Diego Veterans Administration Medical Center, La Jolla, California

Helen S. Mayberg, M.D.
Department of Radiology, Johns Hopkins School of Medicine, Baltimore, Maryland

Robert G. Robinson, M.D.
Department of Psychiatry, University of Iowa, Iowa City, Iowa

Sabine Schlegel, M.D.
Psychiatrische Klinik, Johannes Gutenberg Universitaet-Main, Mainz, Germany

Jeffrey M. Schwartz, M.D.
Department of Psychiatry and Biobehavioral Sciences, The Neuropsychiatric Institute, University of California, Los Angeles, Los Angeles, California

Sergio E. Starkstein, M.D.
Department of Psychiatry and Behavioral Sciences, Johns Hopkins School of Medicine, Baltimore, Maryland

Martin P. Szuba, M.D.
Department of Psychiatry and Biobehavioral Sciences, The Neuropsychiatric Institute, University of California, Los Angeles, Los Angeles, California

Introduction to the Progress in Psychiatry Series

The Progress in Psychiatry Series is designed to capture in print the excitement that comes from assembling a diverse group of experts from various locations to examine in detail the newest information about a developing aspect of psychiatry. This series emerged as a collaboration between the American Psychiatric Association's (APA) Scientific Program Committee and the American Psychiatric Press, Inc. Great interest is generated by a number of the symposia presented each year at the APA annual meeting, and we realized that much of the information presented there, carefully assembled by people who are deeply immersed in a given area, would unfortunately not appear together in print. The symposia sessions at the annual meetings provide an unusual opportunity for experts who otherwise might not meet on the same platform to share their diverse viewpoints for a period of 3 hours. Some new themes are repeatedly reinforced and gain credence, while in other instances disagreements emerge, enabling the audience and now the reader to reach informed decisions about new directions in the field. The Progress in Psychiatry Series allows us to publish and capture some of the best of the symposia and thus provide an in-depth treatment of specific areas that might not otherwise be presented in broader review formats.

Psychiatry is by nature an interface discipline, combining the study of mind and brain, of individual and social environments, of the humane and the scientific. Therefore, progress in the field is rarely linear—it often comes from unexpected sources. Further, new developments emerge from an array of viewpoints that do not necessarily provide immediate agreement but rather expert examination of the issues. We intend to present innovative ideas and data that will enable you, the reader, to participate in this process.

We believe the Progress in Psychiatry Series will provide you with an opportunity to review timely new information in specific fields of interest as they are developing. We hope you find that the excitement of the presentations is captured in the written word and that this book proves to be informative and enjoyable reading.

David Spiegel, M.D.
Series Editor
Progress in Psychiatry Series

Progress in Psychiatry Series Titles

The Borderline: Current Empirical Research (#1)
Edited by Thomas H. McGlashan, M.D.

Premenstrual Syndrome: Current Findings and Future Directions (#2)
Edited by Howard J. Osofsky, M.D., Ph.D., and Susan J. Blumenthal, M.D.

Treatment of Affective Disorders in the Elderly (#3)
Edited by Charles A. Shamoian, M.D.

Post-Traumatic Stress Disorder in Children (#4)
Edited by Spencer Eth, M.D., and Robert S. Pynoos, M.D., M.P.H.

The Psychiatric Implications of Menstruation (#5)
Edited by Judith H. Gold, M.D., F.R.C.P. (C)

Can Schizophrenia Be Localized in the Brain? (#6)
Edited by Nancy C. Andreasen, M.D., Ph.D.

Medical Mimics of Psychiatric Disorders (#7)
Edited by Irl Extein, M.D., and Mark S. Gold, M.D.

Biopsychosocial Aspects of Bereavement (#8)
Edited by Sidney Zisook, M.D.

Psychiatric Pharmacosciences of Children and Adolescents (#9)
Edited by Charles Popper, M.D.

Psychobiology of Bulimia (#10)
Edited by James I. Hudson, M.D., and Harrison G. Pope, Jr., M.D.

Cerebral Hemisphere Function in Depression (#11)
Edited by Marcel Kinsbourne, M.D.

Eating Behavior in Eating Disorders (#12)
Edited by B. Timothy Walsh, M.D.

Tardive Dyskinesia: Biological Mechanisms and Clinical Aspects (#13)
Edited by Marion E. Wolf, M.D., and Aron D. Mosnaim, Ph.D.

Current Approaches to the Prediction of Violence (#14)
Edited by David A. Brizer, M.D., and Martha L. Crowner, M.D.

Treatment of Tricyclic-Resistant Depression (#15)
Edited by Irl L. Extein, M.D.

Depressive Disorders and Immunity (#16)
Edited by Andrew H. Miller, M.D.

Depression and Families: Impact and Treatment (#17)
Edited by Gabor I. Keitner, M.D.

Depression in Schizophrenia (#18)
Edited by Lynn E. DeLisi, M.D.

Biological Assessment and Treatment of Posttraumatic Stress Disorder (#19)
Edited by Earl L. Giller, Jr., M.D., Ph.D.

Personality Disorders: New Perspectives on Diagnostic Validity (#20)
Edited by John M. Oldham, M.D.

Serotonin in Major Psychiatric Disorders (#21)
Edited by Emil F. Coccaro, M.D., and Dennis L. Murphy, M.D.

Amino Acids in Psychiatric Disease (#22)
Edited by Mary Ann Richardson, Ph.D.

Family Environment and Borderline Personality Disorder (#23)
Edited by Paul S. Links, M.D.

Biological Rhythms, Mood Disorders, Light Therapy, and the Pineal Gland (#24)
Edited by Mohammad Shafii, M.D., and Sharon Lee Shafii, R.N., B.S.N.

Treatment Strategies for Refractory Depression (#25)
Edited by Steven P. Roose, M.D., and Alexander H. Glassman, M.D.

Combination Pharmacotherapy and Psychotherapy for Depression (#26)
Edited by Donna Manning, M.D., and Allen J. Frances, M.D.

The Neuroleptic Nonresponsive Patient: Characterization and Treatment (#27)
Edited by Burt Angrist, M.D., and S. Charles Schulz, M.D.

Negative Schizophrenic Symptoms: Pathophysiology and Clinical Implications (#28)
Edited by John F. Greden, M.D., and Rajiv Tandon, M.D.

Neuropeptides and Psychiatric Disorders (#29)
Edited by Charles B. Nemeroff, M.D., Ph.D.

Central Nervous System Peptide Mechanisms in Stress and Depression (#30)
Edited by S. Craig Risch, M.D.

Current Concepts of Somatization: Research and Clinical Perspectives (#31)
Edited by Laurence J. Kirmayer, M.D., F.R.C.P.(C), and James M. Robbins, Ph.D.

Mental Retardation: Developing Pharmacotherapies (#32)
Edited by John J. Ratey, M.D.

Positron-Emission Tomography in Schizophrenia Research (#33)
Edited by Nora D. Volkow, M.D., and Alfred P. Wolf, Ph.D.

Brain Imaging in Affective Disorders (#34)
Edited by Peter Hauser, M.D.

Psychoimmunology Update (#35)
Edited by Jack M. Gorman, M.D., and Robert M. Kertzner, M.D.

Introduction

The rapid development of brain imaging technology in the 1980s has been at the forefront of unprecedented technical advances in brain research and has contributed greatly to a concurrent renaissance of research in psychiatry. Recent progress in our understanding of the brain as it relates to human behavior has directly paralleled these technical advances. Brain imaging has allowed the study of neuroanatomic and biochemical abnormalities that comprise the pathophysiologic processes underlying the symptom picture of psychiatric illnesses, has served to bridge the gap between brain and behavior, and has contributed to the reemergence of neuropsychiatry. Future applications of brain imaging techniques offer the promise of redefining psychiatric illnesses previously conceptualized as functional and of changing irrevocably the method of clinical psychiatric assessment.

Brain imaging techniques can be grouped into structural and functional techniques. Structural techniques permit visualization of brain structure or morphology and include computed tomography (CT) and magnetic resonance imaging (MRI). Functional techniques include brain electrical activity mapping (BEAM), positron-emission tomography (PET), and single photon emission computed tomography (SPECT). BEAM is a technique that utilizes computerized tomographic techniques to display data derived from electroencephalograph (EEG) recordings of brain electrical activity. PET and SPECT permit the study of brain metabolism and cerebral blood flow and also allow the study of neurotransmitter receptor activity or concentration in the brain.

Before we begin to utilize fully a new generation of scanning technology, it may be prudent first to pause and reevaluate the design and methodology of past efforts. This may permit consensus on the methods of measurement employed or on clinical variables that affect brain morphology and function. Historically, neurohistologic staining techniques developed at the turn of the 20th century were greeted by psychiatrists with the same excitement and anticipation as brain imaging is today. After early successes in characterizing neuropathologic abnormalities of certain diseases such as Alzheimer's disease, enthusiasm for the new technique waned. Neurohistology was complicated by several confounding variables secondary to death and tissue fixation and limited to the study of deceased, therefore predominantly elderly patients. Neurohistologic techniques as a method of understanding psychiatric illness were supplanted by the then evolving theories of psychoanalysis.

Although numerous studies in schizophrenia have described neuropathologic changes, no definitive conclusions have been made regarding either the exact nature or the gross anatomic location of these neuropathologic abnormalities. Of interest, neuropathologic investigations in the affective disorders have been largely neglected, although the few neuropathologic studies of schizophrenia that included a comparison group of affective patients have found no significant differences between diagnostic groups. It has been suggested that the reason for this inattention to affective illness relates to the lifetime course of these disorders. Unlike schizophrenia, which has a chronic and progressive course, thereby suggesting a structural brain lesion with sequelae, the affective disorders are typically cyclical with periods of complete remission between episodes of illness. In addition, the pharmacologic treatment of the affective disorders has, in general, proved more effective than that of schizophrenia. Perhaps for these reasons, research in the affective disorders has focused on pharmacologic, biochemical, and neuroendocrine aspects of the illness.

It has been with this bias toward schizophrenia that psychiatrists have entered the age of brain imaging technology. Since the first CT scan study of psychiatric patients by Johnstone in 1976, the predominant focus of structural brain imaging research has been on schizophrenia. Initial studies described lateral ventricular enlargement in schizophrenic patients when compared to control subjects. This has been the most consistent finding, although third ventricle enlargement, cortical and cerebellar atrophy, and abnormalities of cerebral asymmetry and brain tissue density have also been reported. Although fewer in number, studies of patients with affective disorder have uncovered structural brain abnormalities identical to those of schizophrenic patients and thus have raised the question of the specificity of these abnormalities to a particular psychiatric illness. Only a portion of patients in either diagnostic group show ventricular enlargement or other abnormalities. Subsequent CT scan studies in both schizophrenia and the affective disorders have concentrated on understanding the underlying pathophysiologic mechanisms responsible for these abnormalities and on identification and characterization of specific subgroups. Although structural brain abnormalities have correlated with various clinical variables, including treatment response, cognitive impairment, symptomatology, neuroendocrine status, and demographic data, researchers have seldom considered more than a few of these variables simultaneously and there has been no consensus regarding which clinical variables might be associated with which structural brain changes. The observation of structural brain abnormalities in the affective disorders provides justification for the utilization of the new generation of brain imaging technology to elucidate these abnormalities and thereby to suggest possible mechanisms underlying the production of affective symptomatology.

A distinction has been made between primary affective disorders and affective disorders secondary to central nervous system insult with the result that secondary affective disorders in particular can be expected to have demonstrable brain pathology. These secondary affective disorders are important to consider for several reasons. They challenge the theory that a fixed structural lesion can never lead to an episodic illness. They thus provide further justification for structural and functional imaging studies in primary affective disorders. CT scan studies of poststroke patients and MRI studies of multiple sclerosis and temporal lobe epilepsy patients with secondary affective disorder involving known brain lesions offer unique opportunities for assessing relationships between lesion location and the presence or quality of mood disorder. The secondary affective disorders can also be useful as a model to study the effect of focal structural lesions on metabolism and receptor activity of brain regions distant from the lesion site. MRI and PET technology enables researchers to study possible structural and functional abnormalities in the primary affective disorders and make comparisons with structure-function correlations demonstrated in certain secondary affective disorders. It may become possible to distinguish subgroups within the primary affective disorder population who reveal identifiable lesions. This would challenge the concept of primary affective disorder as a purely "mental" phenomenon independent of brain structure or mechanism.

This volume has been written to give the reader a basic understanding of several brain imaging techniques employed in the delineation of brain structure and function in primary and secondary affective disorders. It is a compilation of five investigators' most recent findings in this field and, as such, is not meant as a comprehensive survey.

In the first three chapters, the basic principles and methodological issues involving CT, MRI, and PET techniques, respectively, are described. Studies utilizing each of these techniques in patients with primary affective disorders are discussed. In Chapter 1, Dr. Sabine Schlegel discusses the methodological and topographical aspects of ventricular and density measurements in CT scan studies of patients with primary affective disorders and provides a review of these studies over the past decade. As well, she provides a summary of the most important findings of her own very meticulous studies. In Chapter 2, I review the basic principles of MRI technology and discuss methodological issues in structural brain imaging studies. This is followed by an overview of MRI research in the primary affective disorders. In Chapter 3, Drs. Guze, Baxter, Szuba, and Schwartz explain the general principles of PET technology and demonstrate how this technique has been utilized to study brain metabolism and receptor-ligand interactions in primary affective disorders.

Chapters 4 and 5 focus on brain imaging studies in two related subgroups within the affective disorders spectrum: elderly patients with a mood disorder postulated to be associated with the insidious cerebrovascular changes accompanying old age and patients with an affective syndrome secondary to a focal lesion caused by cerebrovascular accident. In Chapter 4, Dr. Coffey summarizes his MRI findings of structural brain abnormalities in elderly depressed patients and discusses their potential clinical and pathophysiologic significance. In Chapter 5, Drs. Bryer, Starkstein, Mayberg, and Robinson describe how brain lesions in patients with cerebral infarction can be localized and quantified with CT and correlated with the clinical presentation of a mood disorder. They then describe how PET can be utilized to examine the relationship between structural lesions and neuroreceptor imaging of the brain. Chapter 6, written by Drs. Dupont and Jeste, integrates the research findings of the preceding chapters and speculates about the clinical implications of brain imaging research in the affective disorders.

In conclusion, researchers now have the potential, using the new generation of brain imaging technology, to examine specific brain regions of interest in the affective disorders and to understand the underlying pathophysiologic mechanisms responsible for the production of affective symptomatology. The initial observation of structural brain abnormalities in CT scan studies of patients with primary and secondary affective disorders has provided the justification for MRI and PET imaging studies that permit a more precise investigational approach. The task at hand is to design studies that adequately utilize the new technology and that examine the association between structural brain changes and the neuroendocrine, neurochemical, and/or probable genetic abnormalities found in the affective disorders. It is hoped that clinical interventions will benefit from the new insights provided by brain imaging research. This new technology should improve both patient assessment and treatment. Together with personal attention, psychopharmacologic skill, and psychological support, these new methods will provide creative and effective approaches to patients with affective disorder.

This book could not have been written without contributions of Drs. Baxter, Bryer, Coffey, Dupont, Guze, Jeste, Mayberg, Robinson, Schlegel, Schwartz, Starkstein, and Szuba. I also would like to thank Drs. Post and Altschuler and the staff of the Biologic Psychiatry Branch, National Institute of Mental Health; Sandra Boek for her legal assistance; the staff of the American Psychiatric Press; and Jirina, Susi, and Walter Hauser for their ever-present support of my career goals. Particular thanks to Dr. Mary V. Seeman, who continues to be a source of inspiration.

Peter Hauser, M.D.

REFERENCE

Johnstone EC, Crow TJ, Frith CD, et al: Cerebral ventricular size and cognitive impairment in chronic schizophrenia. Lancet 2:924–926, 1976

Chapter 1

Computed Tomography in Affective Disorders

Sabine Schlegel, M.D.

The search for the cause of "melancholia" began more than 2,000 years ago and has concentrated on the study of the brain. The difference between the two sides of the brain was noted nearly 2,400 years ago when the Athenian physician Diocles proposed "that there are two brains in the head: the left one which gives understanding, and the right one which provides sense perception" (Lockhorst 1982).

In 1651, Robert Burton wrote in his famous book, *The Anatomy of Melancholy*, that he agreed with Hippocrates, Galen, and Arabian physicians that melancholia was located in the brain; unlike them, however, he did not think it was caused by ventricular obstruction. Italian physicians of the Renaissance considered deep structures in the brain to be responsible for melancholia. During the 19th century, French neuropsychiatrists suggested encephalitis as the possible cause of affective illness. In 1886, neuropsychiatrist Mairet described circumscribed lesions in the inferior aspects of the temporal lobes from which he thought depressive ideas originated (Berrios 1985).

During the 20th century, neuropathologic and neuroradiologic investigations of depression have been relatively neglected compared to those of schizophrenia and dementia. The first pneumoencephalographic examinations of patients with cyclothymia revealed no abnormalities of the ventricular system (Jacobi and Winkler 1927). Later studies found increased ventricular size only in patients with "residual" symptoms after remission (Huber 1957) or those with severe chronicity (Nagy 1963).

Computed tomography (CT) of the brain offered for the first time a noninvasive method for imaging not only the ventricles but also various other brain structures. In the following section, I review studies of CT in affective disorders with special regard to clinical features.

CT STUDIES COMPARING AFFECTIVE PATIENTS AND CONTROLS

Most CT studies have investigated only the ventricular brain ratio (VBR) as measured by planimetric techniques. The VBR is defined as the area of the lateral ventricles divided by the total area of the brain and multiplied by 100 (Synek and Reuben 1976). To limit the influence of measurement on results in my team's studies, we applied three different techniques of VBR measurements.

Following the guidelines of Zatz and Jernigan (1983), all measurements were made on the same CT scanner under identical window settings on the viewing console. With planimetric VBR (VBR_{plan}) (Figure 1-1), the ventricular area and the total brain area were outlined three times and the mean of three measurements were calculated.

To avoid the difficulties in visually defining ventricular borders by using planimetric measurements, two densitometric methods were additionally applied. By CT different brain structures can be discriminated due to small absorption differences. Correspondingly, attenuation values can be measured in Hounsfield Units (HU), which

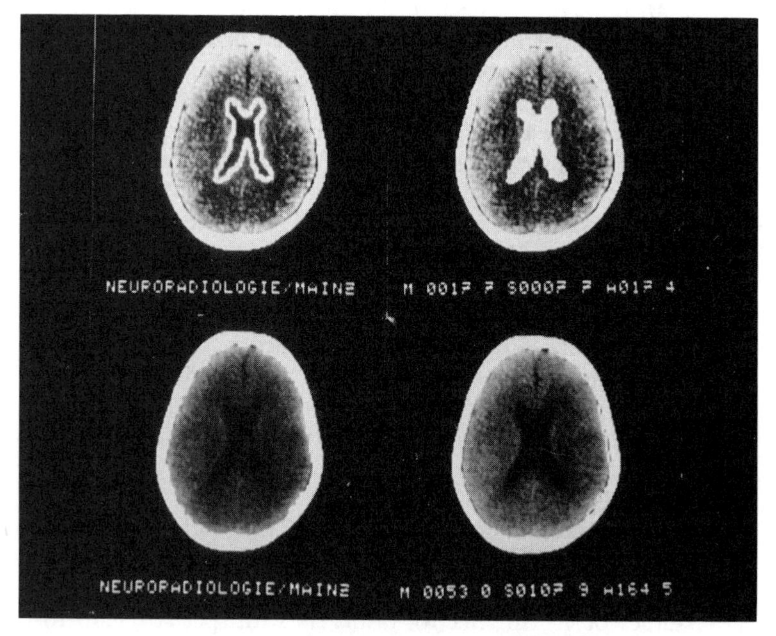

Figure 1-1. Ventricular brain ratio planimetric (VBR_{plan}).

assessed the density of various tissues: water is defined as 0 HU, cerebrospinal fluid (CSF) as 0–5 HU, fat and air below 0 HU, brain as 20–40 HU, and bone above 90 HU. By the densitometric method, all pixels corresponding to CSF were automatically counted in a given region of interest. Due to the surrounding brain tissue, the CSF spaces of the ventricle have a range between 0 and 25 HU. Therefore, the first time, a rectangle was projected on the ventricles and all pixels between 0 and 25 HU were counted in cm^2 (VBR_{25}), as demonstrated in Figure 1-2. The second time, all pixels between 0 and 20 HU were counted (Figure 1-3). The brain area was measured in the same way using a projection of a rectangle counting a density range of 0–80 HU, which corresponds to brain tissue and CSF spaces.

As shown in Table 1-1, several investigators have described larger VBRs in patients with affective disorders compared to controls (Dolan et al. 1986; Kolbeinsson et al. 1986; Luchins et al. 1984; Nasrallah et al. 1982, 1985; Pearlson and Veroff 1981; Pearlson et al. 1984a; Scott et al. 1983; Shima et al. 1984; Targum et al. 1983). As shown in Table 1-2, other investigators could not find such differences (Dewan et al. 1988a; Iacono et al. 1988; Kellner et al. 1983; Schlegel

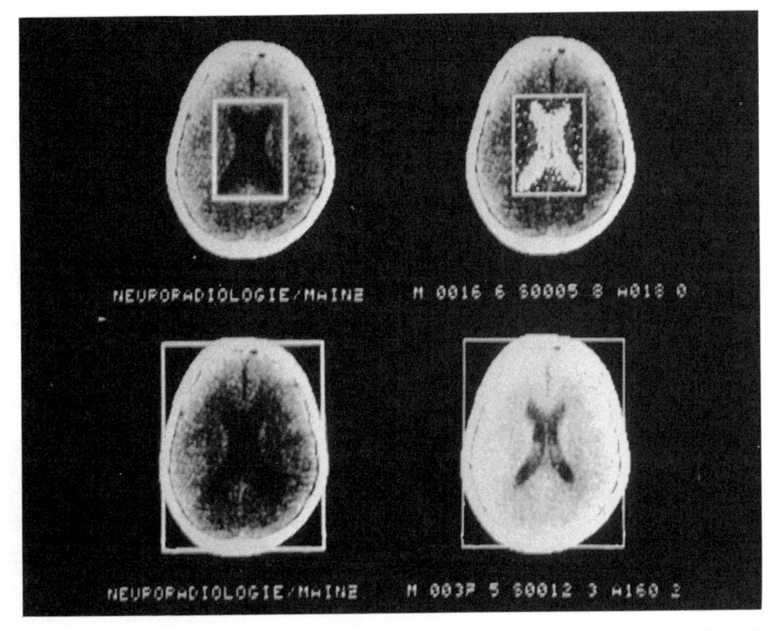

Figure 1-2. Ventricular brain ratio densitometric, all pixels between 0 and 25 HU (VBR_{25}).

and Kretzschmar 1987a; Weinberger et al. 1982). Tables 1-1 and 1-2 show that type of CT scanner, sex ratio, diagnostic systems, age, and selection of controls cannot account for divergent results. Furthermore, the tables demonstrate a wide range of VBR values for patients and controls, making a direct comparison between different studies impossible.

A much smaller number of studies have examined CSF spaces other than the lateral ventricles. Studies have included measurement of the third ventricular width, the anterior horn width, the Huckman number (the sum of the frontal horn and the bicaudate distance), the frontal horn index (the frontal horn distance divided by the outer diameter of the skull), and interhemispheric and Sylvian fissures.

Studies of the third ventricle (Table 1-3) have described slight enlargement in patients older than 50 years (Tanaka et al. 1982) as well as significantly increased width in younger patients (Dewan et al. 1988a; Schlegel and Kretzchmar 1987a) compared to controls. Iacono et al. (1988) could demonstrate an enlarged third ventricle in younger depressed patients only in comparison to medically ill controls, but not in comparison to healthy controls.

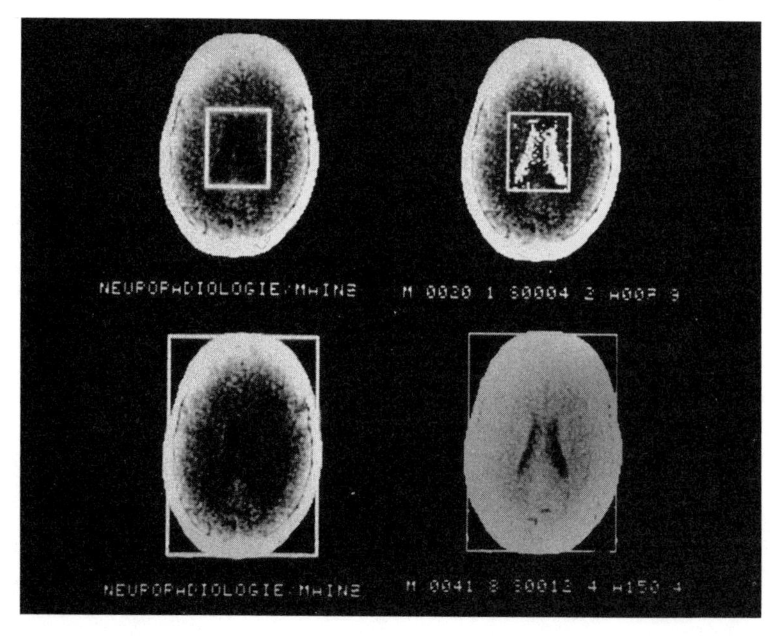

Figure 1-3. Ventricular brain ratio densitometric, all pixels between 0 and 20 HU (VBR_{20}).

Significant differences have also been described for the maximum width of the right anterior horn (Tanaka et al. 1982), the Huckman number, and the frontal horn index (Schlegel and Kretzschmar 1987a).

Tanaka et al. (1982) described a significant widening of the interhemispheric and Sylvian fissures in manic-depressive patients over 49 years of age. Ratings of cerebral sulcal and fissure size have shown that depressed patients had a greater amount of sulcal widening, especially in the frontal and temporal areas (Dolan et al. 1986). Kolbeinsson et al. (1986) also reported sulcal, Sylvian, and interhemispheric fissures widening.

Other authors did not find differences between patients and controls in the Sylvian fissure width (Schlegel and Kretzschmar 1987a), the interhemispheric fissure width (Dewan et al. 1988a; Schlegel and Kretzschmar 1987a), or global atrophy scores (Dewan et al. 1988a; Iacono et al. 1988).

The prevalence of vermian atrophy has been reported to be greater in patients with affective disorders compared with controls (Lippman et al. 1982; Nasrallah et al. 1981; Weinberger et al. 1982).

CT STUDIES COMPARING AFFECTIVE AND SCHIZOPHRENIC PATIENTS

Rieder et al. (1983) compared ventricular size, sulcal prominence, and cerebellar atrophy of bipolar patients with chronic schizophrenic and chronic schizoaffective patients. After age correction, they did not find significant differences across diagnostic groups. Despite the fact that patients with affective disorders did not differ from controls, in contrast to the schizophrenic patients, Weinberger et al. (1982) found no significant differences in ventricular size between the schizophreniform or the chronic schizophrenic groups and the affective disorder group.

CLINICAL VARIABLES

The following clinical variables have been examined in patients with affective disorders:

Unipolar Versus Bipolar Illness

Neither VBR values (Dolan et al. 1985; Schlegel and Kretzschmar 1987a) nor linear measurements of outer and inner CSF spaces differed between unipolar and bipolar patients (Schlegel and Kretzschmar 1987a).

Table 1-1. Significant differences between patients and control subjects in ventricular brain ratio (VBR)

Study and scanner used	*n*	Sex		Diagnosis	Age (yr)	VBR (mean ± SD)	
		Male	Female			Patients	Controls
Pearlson and Veroff (1981) AS&E 500	P: 16 MC: 35	+ ?	+ ?	DSM-III: bipolar MDE + delusional	16–50	6.5 ± 3.3	3.6 ± 2.6
Nasrallah et al. (1982) EMI 1005	P: 24 MC: 27	24 27	0 0	DSM-III: mania	P: 31 C: 28	7.5 ± 3.2	4.5 ± 2.6
Scott et al. (1983) EMI 1010	P: 10 MC: 10	? ?	? ?	DSM-III: MDE + delusional	P: 39.8 C: 39.7	9.4 ± 3.4	4.2 ± 2.9
Targum et al. (1983) EMI 1005/ EMI 1010	P: 38 MC: 26	10 13	28 13	DSM-III: 9 bipolar + 29 unipolar P: 20;NP: 18	P: 30.6 C: 30.5	P: 5.1 ± 3.3 NP: 3.6 ± 2.0	2.9 ± 2.9
Pearlson et al. (1984a) AS&E 500	P: 27 HC: 27	12 12	15 15	DSM-III: bipolar	P: 30.8 C: 30.7	6.6 ± 3.4	4.7 ± 2.1
Luchins et al. (1984) EMI 1005/ SOMATOM II	P: 22 MC: 62	? ?	? ?	RDC: 14 depressive 6 manic 2 schizoaffective	P: 18–59 C: 32.8–38.4	4.5 ± 2.7	3.0 ± 2.3

Shima et al. (1984) EMI 1010/ HITACHI-CTHF	P: 46 C: 46	9 16	37 30	DSM-III: 44 MDE 2 bipolar	P: 53 (25–77) C: 52 (27–78)	11.2 ± 3.5	9.1 ± 2.4
Nasrallah et al. (1985) EMI 1005	P: 19 MC: 27	19 27	0 0	DSM-III: manic/bipolar	P: 31.8 C: 28.7	7.5 ± 3.2	4.5 ± 2.6
Dolan et al. (1985) EMI 1010	P: 108 HC: 52	34 15	74 37	RDC: 74 bipolar 27 unipolar	P: 55.2 C: 54.0	7.2 ± 4.6	5.6 ± 3.3
Kolbeinsson et al. (1986) EMI 5005	P(EC): 22 P: 19 HC: 16	4 5 2	18 14 14	ICD-9	P(EC): 55.1 P: 54.1 HC: 51.9	10.3 ± 1.8 9.5 ± 1.9	8.4 ± 1.5

Note. P = patients. MC = medical controls. HC = healthy controls. C = controls. NP = nonpatients. EC = electroconvulsive therapy. MDE = major depressive episode. RDC = Research Diagnostic Criteria. ICD-9 = International Classification of Diseases, 9th Revision (World Health Organization 1977). + = included in study, but numbers were not specified. ? = data were not reported.

Table 1-2. No significant differences between patients and control subjects in ventricular brain ratio (VBR)

Study and scanner used	*n*	Sex		Diagnosis	Age (yr)	VBR (mean ± SD)	
		Male	Female			Patients	Controls
Weinberger et al. (1982) EMI 1010	P: 23 MC: 26	8 13	15 13	DSM-III	P: 30.3 C: 30.3	3.8 ± 2.9	2.9 ± 2.9
Kellner et al. (1983) EMI 1005/ EMI 1010	P: 10 MC: 12	? ?	? ?	RDC: MDE or bipolar	P: 43.5 (27–69) C: age matched?	5.5 ± 2.7	5.5 ± 2.8
Schlegel and Kretzschmar (1987a) EMI 1010	P: 60 MC: 60	20 20	40 40	DSM-III: MDE 33 unipolar 22 bipolar 5 schizoaffective (RDC)	P: 45.2 C: 45.2	7.4 ± 2.4[a] 6.9 ± 3.7[b] 3.7 ± 3.0[c]	6.9 ± 2.6[a] 6.9 ± 3.2[b] 3.3 ± 2.3[c]
Dewan et al. (1988a) GE 8800	P: 26 MC: 22	19 12	7 10	DSM-III bipolar	P: 32.7 C: 31.1	6.9 ± 2.9	6.3 ± 1.9
Iacono et al. (1988) Somatom DRZ	P(bipolar): 18 P(MDE): 16 MC: 30 HC: 44	9 11 13 29	9 5 17 15	DSM-III	P(bipolar): 26.1 P(MDE): 22.6 MC: 22.9 HC: 23.2	6.2 ± 1.9 6.4 ± 3.0	 5.8 ± 2.5 6.4 ± 2.8

Note. P = patients. MC = medical controls. HC = healthy controls. RDC = Research Diagnostic Criteria. MDE = major depressive episode.

[a]Ventricular brain ratio planimetric (VBR_{plan}). [b]Ventricular brain ratio, all pixels between 0–25 HU (VBR_{25}). [c]Ventricular brain ratio, all pixels between 0–20 HU (VBR_{20}).

Table 1-3. Studies of the third ventricle: differences between patients and control subjects

Study and scanner used	*n*	Sex		Diagnosis	Age (yr)	Third ventricle (mean ± SD)	
		Male	Female			Patients	Controls
Tanaka et al.	P: 40	15	25	31 unipolar	P<49: 35.6	7.9 ± 1.4	
(1982)	MC: 40	19	21	9 bipolar[a]	P>49: 62.8	8.8 ± 2.0	
					MC<49: 35.6		7.6 ± 1.9
					MC>49: 63.3		7.3 ± 1.7
Schlegel and Kretzschmar	P: 60	20	40	DSM-III	P: 45.2	4.3 ± 1.9[b]	3.5 ± 1.1
(1987a)	MC: 60	20	40		C: 45.2		
EMI 1010							
Dewan et al.	P: 26	19	7	DSM-III:	P: 32.7	4.5 ± 1.1[b]	4.0 ± 0.9
(1988a)	MC: 22	12	10	bipolar	C: 31.1		
GE 8800							
Iacono et al.	P(bipolar): 18	9	9	DSM-III	P(bipolar): 26.1	3.3 ± 1.0	
(1988)	P(MDE): 16	11	5		P(MDE): 22.6	3.6 ± 0.9[c]	
Somatom DRZ	MC: 30	13	17		MC: 22.9		3.0 ± 0.9
	HC: 44	29	15		HC: 23.2		3.5 ± 1.1

Note. P = patients. MC = medical controls. C = controls. HC = healthy controls. MDE = major depressive episode.
[a]Diagnostic scale was not specified. [b]Significant differences. [c]Significant differences only compared with medical controls.

"Endogenous" Versus "Nonendogenous" Depression

To compare "endogenous" and "nonendogenous" patients, six different diagnostic systems were applied: 1) DSM-III (American Psychiatric Association 1980); 2) Research Diagnostic Criteria (Spitzer et al. 1978); 3) Newcastle Scale 1 (Bech et al. 1980; Carney et al. 1965); 4) Newcastle Scale 2 (Bech et al. 1980; Gurney 1971); 5) Taylor-Abrams Criteria (Berner et al. 1983; Taylor et al. 1981); and 6) Vienna Research Criteria (Berner et al. 1983). No significant differences between the two types of patients were detected in VBR values (Schlegel et al. 1989b).

Psychotic Versus Nonpsychotic Patients

A tendency to greater VBR values in psychotic patients compared with nonpsychotic patients has been reported; (Luchins and Meltzer 1983; Schlegel and Kretzschmar 1987a; Schlegel et al. 1989b; Targum et al. 1983) (Table 1-4). When patients with the smallest VBR were compared with patients with the largest VBR, differences were not obvious (Luchins et al. 1984) or were even undetectable (Dewan et al. 1988b; Nasrallah et al. 1985; Pearlson et al. 1984a) (Table 1-5).

Comparing psychotic patients with individually age- and sex-matched controls, psychotic patients had a wider diameter of the third ventricle, the Huckman number, and the frontal horn index (Schlegel and Kretzschmar 1987a), whereas nonpsychotic patients did not differ from sex- and age-matched controls in any CT variable (Schlegel and Kretzschmar 1987a).

In sum, at least from my team's data, psychotic patients had wider CSF spaces than nonpsychotic patients. Whether ventricular enlargement is a risk factor that potentiates the development of psychotic symptoms or whether it results from the psychotic process remains unclear.

Severity of Illness

Little attention has been paid to the association between severity of depression and CT measurements. Luchins et al. (1984) could not find a relationship between the score of the Global Assessment Scale (GAS) (Spitzer et al. 1973) and VBR measurements. However, in drug-free depressed patients, significant correlations between VBR values such as the diameter of the third ventricle with the scores of the Brief Psychiatric Rating Scale (BPRS) (Overall and Gorham 1962), the GAS, the Bech-Rafaelsen Melancholia Scale (BRMS) (Bech and Rafaelsen 1980), and the Scale for the Assessment of Negative Symptoms (SANS) (Andreasen et al. 1982) were detected

Table 1-4. Psychotic depression versus nonpsychotic depression (mean ± SD)

Study	Measure	Psychotic	*n*	Nonpsychotic	*n*	*P*<
Targum et al. (1983)	VBR	5.1 ± 3.3	20	3.6 ± 2.0	18	.10
Luchins and Meltzer (1983)	VBR	4.9 ± 2.5	9(?)	3.4 ± 2.4	9	.15
Schlegel and Kretzschmar (1987a)	VBR_{plan}	8.4 ± 2.8	19	6.8 ± 1.9	34	.05
	VBR_{25}	8.5 ± 3.9	19	6.1 ± 3.3	34	.05
	VBR_{20}	5.0 ± 3.6	19	3.0 ± 2.2	34	.05
	Third ventricle	4.9 ± 2.2	22	3.9 ± 1.6	38	NS
	FH+CC	47.0 ± 7.0	22	43.0 ± 6.0	38	.05
	FHot/FH	3.4 ± 0.3	22	3.6 ± 0.4	38	NS
	SFr	4.0 ± 2.1	22	3.5 ± 1.5	38	NS
	SFl	3.7 ± 1.9	22	3.3 ± 1.5	38	NS
	IF	3.2 ± 1.9	22	2.6 ± 1.6	38	NS
Schlegel et al. (1989b)	VBR_{plan}	6.4 ± 2.7	10	5.0 ± 2.9	34	NS
	VBR_{25}	7.9 ± 3.7	10	5.8 ± 4.2	34	NS
	VBR_{20}	4.6 ± 2.9	10	3.1 ± 3.0	34	NS
	Third ventricle	4.8 ± 1.2[a]	10	3.8 ± 1.3	34	.05
	FH+CC	45.9 ± 3.3[a]	10	44.1 ± 6.7	34	NS
	FHot/FH	3.3 ± 0.2	10	3.5 ± 0.5	34	NS
	SFr	5.7 ± 1.7	10	3.8 ± 1.7	34	.05
	SFl	5.4 ± 1.8	10	3.3 ± 1.7	34	.01
	IF	3.0 ± 1.8	10	2.9 ± 1.8	34	NS

Note. VBR = ventricular brain ratio. VBR_{plan} = ventricular brain ratio planimetric. VBR_{25} = ventricular brain ratio, all pixels between 0–25 HU. VBR_{20} = ventricular brain ratio, all pixels between 0–20 HU. FH+CC = Huckman number (sum of frontal horn and bicaudate distance). FHot/FH = frontal horn index. SFr = Sylvian fissure right. SFl = Sylvian fissure left. IF = interhemispheric fissure. NS = not significant.

[a]Significantly greater values in psychotic patients compared to age- and sex-matched controls.

(Schlegel et al. 1989b). Item analyses of the BRMS revealed that ventricle size was most clearly associated with verbal, motor, emotional, and intellectual retardation and depressed mood, but not with anxiety or somatic complaints. The greater consideration of retardation items on the BRMS compared to the Hamilton Rating Scale for Depression (Hamilton 1960) might explain why the Hamilton scale showed no significant correlations with any CT parameter.

An association between VBR and negative symptoms, assessed by the Krawiecka rating scale (Krawiecka et al. 1977) during euthymic state in bipolar patients, was detected by correlation analyses between VBR versus negative symptoms (Pearlson et al. 1984b) but not by comparing patients with the smallest versus the largest VBR (Pearlson et al. 1984b). Similarly, Dewan et al. (1988b) could not find differences in the SANS (during euthymic state) if patients with VBR 1 standard deviation (SD) above the control group were compared with patients who had a VBR below 1 SD of the controls.

Cognition

VBR was not associated with cognitive dysfunctioning as measured by the Mini-Mental State (MMS) (Dewan et al. 1988b; Folstein et al. 1975; Nasrallah et al. 1985; Pearlson et al. 1984a; Schlegel et al. 1988) or the Wechsler Adult Intelligence Scale (Dewan et al. 1988b; Wechsler 1981). An impairment on the Halstead-Reitan Neuropsychological Test Battery (Reitan 1979) was related to larger VBR

Table 1-5. Psychotic symptoms in patients with larger versus smaller ventricular brain ratio (VBR)

Pearlson et al. (1984a)	No difference between 6 patients with largest versus 6 patients with smallest VBR on delusional symptoms (bipolars)
Luchins et al. (1984)	6 patients with VBR > 1 SD (SD of controls); all patients had psychotic symptoms 6 patients with VBR < 1 SD (SD of controls); 50% of the patients had psychotic symptoms (*P* < .06)
Nasrallah et al. (1985)	No difference between 6 patients with VBR > 2 SD versus 13 patients with VBR < 2 SD (SD of controls) for presence of delusions in manic patients
Dewan et al. (1988b)	17 patients with VBR < 1 SD (SD of controls) versus 9 patients with VBR > 1 SD; no significant differences in the occurrence of delusions or hallucinations

Note. SD = standard deviation.

(Dewan et al. 1988b; Kellner et al. 1986). Dewan et al. (1988b) compared patients with smaller VBRs to patients with larger VBRs (defined, respectively, as 1 SD below and 1 SD above the SD of the control group); patients with larger VBRs had a significantly greater Halstead-Reitan impairment index, but did not differ in average impairment rating or percentage of impaired ratings from patients with smaller VBRs. Kellner et al. (1986) found a significant correlation between the number of Halstead-Reitan category test errors and the VBR.

Previous Medications

Dolan et al. (1985, 1986) could not find a relationship between the type of previous treatment or length of treatment with phenothiazines, tricyclic antidepressants monoamine oxidase inhibitors, lithium, or benzodiazepines with VBR or sulcal widening. Comparing patients with the largest VBRs to those with the smallest VBRs, no differences were found in current drug exposure (Pearlson et al. 1984a). Previous treatment with lithium, antidepressants, or neuroleptics was not related to VBR (Luchins et al. 1984). VBR was also not associated with responsiveness to lithium (Dewan et al. 1988b) nor to full response to any drug treatment (Nasrallah et al. 1985). Patients with previous or concurrent lithium therapy did not differ in different VBR measurements, various linear CT parameters, or the Sylvian and interhemispheric fissure measures from patients without lithium treatment (Schlegel and Kretzschmar 1987a).

Electroconvulsive Therapy (ECT)

No relationship was found between ECT and VBR (Dolan et al. 1985; Kolbeinsson et al. 1986; Nasrallah et al. 1982, 1985; Pearlson et al. 1985). The finding that patients with a history of ECT had a greater frequency of sulcal widening in parietal and occipital areas, independent of the number of treatments with ECT (Dolan et al. 1986), could not be confirmed by Kolbeinsson et al. (1986).

Family History of Psychiatric Illness

Family history of psychiatric illness was not related to VBR values (Dewan et al. 1988b; Dolan et al. 1985; Nasrallah et al. 1985; Pearlson et al. 1985), sulcal widening (Dewan et al. 1988b; Dolan et al. 1986), or third ventricle size (Dewan et al. 1988b).

Unemployment

Pearlson et al. (1984b) found an association between unemployment and increased VBR since only unemployed patients differed significantly from controls. In contrast, comparing patients with a VBR 1 SD above controls versus patients with a VBR 1 SD below controls revealed no difference in the percentage of employment (Dewan et al. 1988b).

Course of Illness

Table 1-6 shows that most studies have found no relationship between VBR and duration of illness, number of episodes, episodes per year, number of hospitalizations, hospitalizations per year, and length

Table 1-6. Relationship between clinical data and ventricular brain ratio (VBR)

Duration since first episode	
Pearlson et al. (1984a)	NS
Nasrallah et al. (1985)	NS
Schlegel and Kretzschmar (1987a)	NS
Dewan et al. (1988b)	NS
Roy-Byrne et al. (1988)	NS
Episodes	
Pearlson et al. (1984b)	+
Schlegel and Kretzschmar (1987a)	NS
Dewan et al. (1988b)	NS
Roy-Byrne et al. (1988)	NS
Episodes/year	
Pearlson et al. (1984b)	NS
Nasrallah et al. (1985)	+
Schlegel and Kretzschmar (1987a)	NS
Dewan et al. (1988b)	NS
Roy-Byrne et al. (1988)	NS
Hospitalizations	
Pearlson et al. (1984b)	+
Dolan et al. (1985)	NS
Dewan et al. (1988b)	NS
Roy-Byrne et al. (1988)	NS
Hospitalizations/year	
Nasrallah et al. (1985)	+
Dewan et al. (1988b)	NS
Roy-Byrne et al. (1988)	NS
Length of illness	
Dolan et al. (1985)	NS
Roy-Byrne et al. (1988)	NS

Note. NS = no significant relationship. + = relationship with larger VBR.

of illness. VBR was also not associated with therapy response (Luchins et al. 1984; Nasrallah et al. 1985), or rehospitalization during the year subsequent to the CT examination (Targum et al. 1983). Patients with "residual" syndromes after remission showed an abnormal width of the third ventricle (Gross et al. 1982).

In elderly depressed patients, Jacoby and Levy (1980) found no relationship between ventricle size and treatment response after 3 months, but a higher mortality in patients with greater ventricles was reported after 2 years (Jacoby and Bird 1981). Shima et al. (1984) found that elderly depressed patients with a poorer outcome 9 months after admission had larger VBRs than controls.

Electroencephalogram (EEG)

Manic males (Nasrallah et al. 1985) or bipolar patients (Dewan et al. 1988b) with larger VBRs did not have abnormal EEGs more often than patients with smaller ventricles, but increased third ventricle width was inversely associated with EEG abnormality (Dewan et al. 1988b).

Hypothalamic-Pituitary-Adrenal Axis

Patients with suppression on the dexamethasone suppression test (DST) did not differ from patients without DST suppression in VBR values (Schlegel and Kretzschmar 1987a; Schlegel et al. 1989a; Targum et al. 1983). Baseline 8 A.M. and 4 P.M. postdexamethasone plasma cortisol levels in euthymic bipolar patients did not correlate with VBR (Dewan et al. 1988c). In contrast, free urinary cortisol excretion (Kellner et al. 1983) and mean baseline plasma cortisol levels (nine blood samples between 2 P.M. and 5 P.M.) correlated with VBR values (Schlegel et al. 1989a).

Hypothalamic-Pituitary-Thyroid Axis

Blunted thyroid-stimulating hormone responses to the thyrotropin-releasing hormone stimulation test were not related to VBR (Targum et al. 1983). Johnstone et al. (1986) described an association between VBR and hypothyroidism. However, correlations between triiodothyronine (T3) and thyroxine (T4) values and various ventricle measurements revealed no significant results (Schlegel 1989).

Biochemical Examinations

Larger VBR was associated with low plasma dopamine beta-hydroxylase activity (the enzyme that catalyzes the formation of norepinephrine from dopamine) (Meltzer et al. 1984) and increased ventricular CSF 5-hydroxyindoleacetic acid (the metabolite of 5-hydroxytryptamine) (Standish-Barry et al. 1986), but not with homovanillic acid (the metabolite of dopamine) in the CSF (Standish-Barry et al. 1986).

BRAIN TISSUE DENSITY

Measurements of brain tissue density can provide additional information of structural brain alterations, but depend on the type of CT scanner; the scanner drift from day to day; the size and localization of tissue samples; the size of the ventricles, the brain, the head, and the skull; and bone density (Albert et al. 1984; Coffman and Bloch 1984; Schlegel and Kretzschmar 1987b). These technical conditions might be one reason for controversial results in dementia and schizophrenia since lower density (Albert et al. 1984; Bondareff et al. 1981; Golden et al. 1981), no differences (Wilson et al. 1982), or even higher density (Dewan et al. 1983; George et al. 1981; Pearlson et al. 1981) values were described compared to controls.

In contrast, two studies (Dewan et al. 1988a; Schlegel and Kretzschmar 1987b) that compared controls to patients with affective disorders reported higher density values in patients, but interpreted these findings differently. Schlegel and Kretzschmar revealed higher density values in the left caudate, the left thalamus, the left frontal gray substance, and the right occipital region. When patients were divided into various clinical subgroups, only patients with smaller ventricles had higher density values than controls, whereas patients with greater ventricles than controls showed no differences in density measurements. Because of the inverse correlation between density and ventricular size, higher density values in patients were not considered as an abnormal finding in this study. By contrast, increased density in the right and left caudate and the right and left thalamus in bipolar patients compared to controls was described as an abnormal finding by Dewan et al. The authors found a greater size of the third ventricle in the same group of patients compared to controls, whereas patients with greater ventricles did not differ in brain density from patients with smaller ventricles.

Right-Left Asymmetry

The "normal" interhemispheric differences of brain density (higher density in the left hemisphere than in the right hemisphere) (Coffman and Bloch 1984) were diminished in manic patients (Coffman and Nasrallah 1984). In contrast, Schlegel and Kretzschmar (1987b) found higher left density values in both patients and in controls.

Psychopathology

Psychotic patients had lower density values than nonpsychotic patients, and unipolar patients had lower values than bipolar patients (Schlegel and Kretzschmar 1987b). An inverse correlation was detected between lower density values and the total scores on both the BPRS and BRMS (Schlegel 1989).

Neuroendocrinology

Comparisons between DST suppressors and DST nonsuppressors revealed no significant differences in brain density (Schlegel and Kretzschmar 1987b; Schlegel et al. 1988). No significant correlations were detected between baseline plasma cortisol and density.

SUMMARY

Some, but not all, studies found larger ventricles in patients with affective disorders compared to controls. Increased ventricle size was associated with psychotic symptoms, psychomotor retardation, cognitive impairment on the Halstead-Reitan battery, lower dopamine beta-hydroxylase, higher 5-hydroxyindoleacetic levels, urinary free cortisol excretion, and mean baseline plasma cortisol. The majority of investigations could not find a relationship between ventricle size and family history, DST response, EEG abnormalities, the score of the psychopathology rating scales, previous medication, ECT, duration of illness, number of episodes, frequency of hospitalizations, or therapy response.

CONCLUSION

The value of CT investigations in affective disorders is limited for the following reasons. First, most significant findings are only group mean differences. No individual scan is radiologically abnormal. Second, results are not reproducible. Third, no neuropathologic studies with a primary focus on the neuropathology of affective disorders have as yet been reported (Jeste et al. 1988). Therefore, the pathophysiologic mechanisms underlying purported brain abnormalities in affective disorders remain obscure. Fourth, it is not clear whether CT alterations are a preexisting risk factor for the development of affective disorders (dysgenesis) or the result of the illness (atrophy). Fifth, until now, no clinical implications of CT abnormalities in affective disorders have been noted. Finally, cerebral regions most likely to be associated with affective disorders (i.e., limbic structures) are not measurable by CT, due to artifacts.

In conclusion, CT findings provide only a descriptive approach. Therefore, the biological mechanism remains a matter of speculation. One hypothesis might be that the subtype of psychomotor retarded depression is associated with CT alterations. This hypothesis is supported by 1) the concomitancy of depression in Parkinson's disease; 2) low homovanillic acid levels in retarded depressed patients (for review, see Jimerson 1987); 3) decreased dopamine in the putamen, caudate, and nucleus ruber in postmortem examinations in depressive patients (Birkmayer and Riederer 1988); 4) smaller areas of the caudate in affective disorders compared to schizophrenia or Alzheimer's disease on neuropathologic investigations (Brown et al. 1986); and 5) lower glucose metabolism in the head of the caudate during depression measured by positron-emission tomography (Baxter et al. 1985).

However, there are also arguments against this hypothesis of an association between brain alterations and the dopamine pathway. First, ventricular size was most clearly associated with the concomitant occurrence of retardation and psychotic features (Schlegel et al. 1989b). Second, psychotic symptoms in depression were associated with higher homovanillic acid levels (Sweeny et al. 1978). Third, homovanillic acid levels were not associated with ventricular size (Standish-Barry et al. 1986).

A further hypothesis is a causal relationship between cortisol and ventricular size as suggested by studies in Cushing's disease (Heinz et al. 1977), anorexia nervosa (Krieg et al. 1986, 1988), and steroid hormone treatment (Bentson et al. 1978). All these studies found a reversibility of cerebral "atrophy" once the hormone levels were normalized. In contrast to the above clinical conditions, both the brain alterations and cortisol levels in depression are modest and do not reach clinical significance.

Further speculations on possible relationships with perinatal brain injuries, weight loss, or alcohol intake have been discussed by Nasrallah et al. (1989). Both weight loss and alcohol intake were controlled in patients and controls by Pearlson et al. (1984a) and Dolan et al. (1985) and therefore did not account for the difference in ventricular size.

In summary, present knowledge does not allow conclusive explanations or interpretations of CT alterations in affective disorders.

REFERENCES

Albert M, Naeser MA, Levine HL, et al: CT density numbers in patients with senile dementia of the Alzheimer's type. Arch Neurol 41:1264–1269, 1984

American Psychiatric Association: Diagnostic and Statistical Manual of Mental Disorders, 3rd Edition. Washington, DC, American Psychiatric Association, 1980

Andreasen NC, Olsen SA, Dennert JW, et al: Ventricular enlargement in schizophrenia: relationship to positive and negative symptoms. Am J Psychiatry 139:297–302, 1982

Baxter LR, Phelps ME, Mazziotta JC, et al: Cerebral metabolic rates for glucose in mood disorders. Arch Gen Psychiatry 42:441–447, 1985

Bech P, Rafaelsen OJ: The use of rating scales exemplified by comparison of the Hamilton and the Bech-Rafaelsen melancholia scale. Acta Psychiatr Scand (Suppl) 285:128–146, 1980

Bech P, Gram LF, Reisby N, et al: The WHO depression scale: relationship to the Newcastle scales. Acta Psychiatr Scand 62:140–153, 1980

Bentson JR, Reza M, Winter J, et al: Steroids and apparent cerebral atrophy on computed tomography scans. J Comput Assist Tomogr 2:16–23, 1978

Berner P, Gabriel E, Katschnig H, et al: Diagnostic criteria of schizophrenic and affective disorders. Wien, World Psychiatric Association, 1983

Berrios GE: "Depressive pseudodementia" or "melancholic dementia": a 19th century view. J Neurol Neurosurg Psychiatry 48:393–400, 1985

Birkmayer W, Riederer P: Depression. Köln, Deutscher Ärzte-Verlag, 1988

Bondareff W, Baldy R, Levy R: Quantitative computed tomography in senile dementia. Arch Gen Psychiatry 38:1365–1368, 1981

Brown R, Colter N, Corsellis JAN, et al: Postmortem evidence of structural brain changes in schizophrenia. Arch Gen Psychiatry 43:36–42, 1986

Burton R: The Anatomy of Melancholy. Oxford, 1651

Carney MWP, Roth M, Garside RF: The diagnosis of depressive syndromes and the prediction of ECT response. Br J Psychiatry 121:659–674, 1965

Coffman JA, Bloch S: Interhemispheric differences in regional density of the normal brain. J Psychiatr Res 18:269–275, 1984

Coffman JA, Nasrallah HA: Brain density patterns in schizophrenia and mania. J Affective Disord 6:307–315, 1984

Coffman JA, Nasrallah HA: Relationships between brain density, cortical atrophy and ventriculomegaly in schizophrenia and mania. Acta Psychiatr Scand 72:126–132, 1985

Dewan MJ, Pandurangi AK, Lee SH, et al: Central brain morphology in chronic schizophrenic patients: a controlled CT study. Biol Psychiatry 18:1133–1140, 1983

Dewan MJ, Haldipur CV, Lane EE, et al: Bipolar affective disorder, I: comprehensive quantitative computed tomography. Acta Psychiatr

Scand 77:670–676, 1988a

Dewan MJ, Haldipur CV, Boucher MF, et al: Bipolar affective disorder, II: EEG, neuropsychological, and clinical correlates of CT abnormality. Acta Psychiatr Scand 77:677–682, 1988b

Dewan MJ, Haldipur CV, Boucher MF, et al: Is ventriculomegaly related to hypercortisolemia? Acta Psychiatr Scand 77:230–231, 1988c

Dolan RJ, Colloway SP, Mann AH: Cerebral ventricular size in depressed subjects. Psychol Med 15:873–878, 1985

Dolan RJ, Colloway SP, Thacker PF, et al: The cerebral cortical appearance in depressed subjects. Psychol Med 16:775–779, 1986

Folstein MF, Folstein SE, McHugh PR: Mini-Mental State: a practical method for grading the cognitive state of patients for the clinician. J Psychiatr Res 12:189–198, 1975

George AJ, deLeon MJ, Ferris SH, et al: Parenchymal CT correlates of senile dementia (Alzheimer disease): loss of gray-white matter discriminability. AJNR 2:205–211, 1981

Golden CJ, Graber B, Coffman J, et al: Structural brain deficits in schizophrenia: identification by computed tomographic scan density measurements. Arch Gen Psychiatry 38:1014–1017, 1981

Gross G, Huber G, Schuettler R: Computerized tomography studies on schizophrenic diseases. Archiv fuer Psychiatrie und Nervenkrankheiten 321:519–526, 1982

Gurney C: Diagnostic scales for affective disorders. Proceedings of the Fifth World Congress of Psychiatry, Mexico City, 1971, p 330

Hamilton M: A rating scale for depression. J Neurol Neurosurg Psychiatry 23:56–62, 1960

Heinz ER, Martinez J, Haenggeli A: Reversibility of cerebral atrophy in anorexia nervosa and Cushing's syndrome. J Comput Assist Tomogr 1:415–418, 1977

Huber G: Pneumoencephalographische und psychopathologische Bilder bei endogenen Psychosen. Berlin, Springer-Verlag, 1957

Iacono WG, Smith GN, Moreau M, et al: Ventricular and sulcal size at the onset of psychosis. Am J Psychiatry 145:820–824, 1988

Jacobi W, Winkler H: Encephalographische Studien an Schizophrenen. Archiv fuer Psychiatrie und Nervenkrankheiten 82:208–226, 1927

Jacoby RJ, Bird JM: Computed tomography and the outcome in affective disorder: a follow-up study of elderly patients. Br J Psychiatry 139:288–292, 1981

Jacoby RJ, Levy R: Computed tomography in the elderly, 3: affective disorder. Br J Psychiatry 136:270–275, 1980

Jeste DV, Lohr JB, Goodwin FK: Neuroanatomical studies of major affective disorders: a review and suggestions for further research. Br J Psychiatry 153:444–459, 1988

Jimerson DC: Role of dopamine mechanisms in the affective disorders, in Psychopharmacology: The Third Generation of Progress. Edited by Meltzer, HY. New York, Raven, 1987, pp 505–512

Johnstone EC, Owens DGC, Crow TJ, et al: Hypothyroidism as a correlate of lateral ventricular enlargement in manic-depressive and neurotic illness. Br J Psychiatry 148:317–321, 1986

Kellner CH, Rubinow DR, Gold PW, et al: Relationship of cortisol hypersecretion to brain CT scan alterations in depressed patients. Psychiatry Res 8:191–197, 1983

Kellner CH, Rubinow DR, Post RM: Cerebral ventricular size and cognitive impairment in depression. J Affective Disord 10:215–219, 1986

Kolbeinsson H, Arnaldsson OS, Petursson H, et al: Computed tomographic scans in ECT-patients. Acta Psychiatr Scand 73:28–32, 1986

Krawiecka M, Goldberg D, Vaughan M: A standardized psychiatric assessment scale for rating chronic psychotic patients. Acta Psychiatr Scand 55:299–308, 1977

Krieg JC, Backmund H, Pirke KM: Endocrine, metabolic, and brain morphological abnormalities in patients with eating disorders. International Journal of Eating Disorders 5:999–1005, 1986

Krieg JC, Pirke KM, Lauer C, et al: Endocrine, metabolic, and cranial computed tomographic findings in anorexia nervosa. Biol Psychiatry 23:377–387, 1988

Lippman S, Manshadi M, Baldwin H, et al: Cerebellar vermis dimensions on computerized tomographic scans of schizophrenic and bipolar patients. Am J Psychiatry 139:667–668, 1982

Lockhorst QJC: Classics in neurology. Neurology (NY) 32:762, 1982

Luchins DJ, Meltzer HY: Ventricular size and psychosis in affective disorder. Biol Psychiatry 18:1197–1198, 1983

Luchins DJ, Levine RJ, Meltzer HY: Lateral ventricular size, psychopathology and medication response in the psychoses. Biol Psychiatry 19:29–44, 1984

Meltzer HY, Tong C, Luchins DJ: Serum dopamine-β-hydroxylase activity and lateral ventricular size in affective disorders and schizophrenia. Biol

Psychiatry 19:1395–1402, 1984

Nagy K: Pneumoencephalographische Befunde bei endogenen Psychosen. Nervenarzt 34:543–548, 1963

Nasrallah HA, Jacoby CG, McCalley-Whitters M: Cerebellar atrophy in schizophrenia and mania. Lancet 1:1102, 1981

Nasrallah HA, McCalley-Whitters M, Jacoby CG: Cerebral ventricular enlargement in young manic males: a controlled CT study. J Affective Disord 4:15–19, 1982

Nasrallah HA, McCalley-Whitters M, Pfahl B: Clinical significance of large cerebral ventricles in manic males. Psychiatry Res 13:151–156, 1985

Nasrallah HA, Coffman JA, Olson SC: Structural brain-imaging findings in affective disorders: an overview. Journal of Neuropsychiatry 1:21–67, 1989

Overall JE, Gorham DR: The Brief Psychiatric Rating Scale. Psychol Rep 10:799–812, 1962

Pearlson GD, Veroff AE: Computerized tomographic scan changes in manic-depressive illness. Lancet 2:470, 1981

Pearlson GD, Veroff AE, McHugh PR: The use of computed tomography in psychiatry: recent application to schizophrenia, manic-depressive illness and dementia syndromes. Johns Hopkins Medical Journal 149: 194–202, 1981

Pearlson GD, Garbacz DJ, Tompkins RH, et al: Clinical correlates of lateral ventricular enlargement in bipolar affective disorder. Am J Psychiatry 141:253–256, 1984a

Pearlson GD, Garbacz DJ, Breakey WR, et al: Lateral ventricular enlargement associated with persistent unemployment and negative symptoms in both schizophrenia and bipolar disorder. Psychiatry Res 12:1–9, 1984b

Pearlson GD, Garbacz DJ, Moberg PJ, et al: Symptomatic, familial perinatal and social correlates of computerized axial tomography (CAT) changes in schizophrenics and unipolars. J Nerv Ment Dis 173:42–50, 1985

Reitan RM: Halstead-Reitan Neuropsychological Test Battery. Tucson, AZ, Neuropsychology Laboratory, University of Arizona, 1979

Rieder RO, Mann LS, Weinberger DR, et al: Computed tomographic scans in patients with schizophrenia, schizoaffective, and bipolar disorder. Arch Gen Psychiatry 40:735–739, 1983

Roy-Byrne P, Post R, Kellner C, et al: Ventricular brain ratio and life course of illness in patients with affective disorders. Psychiatry Res 23:277–284, 1988

Schlegel S: CT in Affective Disorders. American Psychiatric Association, San Francisco, CA, 1989

Schlegel S: Brain density in depression: methodological and psychopathological aspects. Acta Psychiatr Scand 78:610–612, 1988

Schlegel S, Kretzschmar K: Computed tomography in affective disorders, part I: ventricular and sulcal measurements. Biol Psychiatry 22:4–14, 1987a

Schlegel S, Kretzschmar K: Computed tomography in affective disorders, part II: brain density. Biol Psychiatry 22:15–23, 1987b

Schlegel S, Maier W, Philipp M, et al: The association between psychopathological aspects and CT measurements in affective disorders. Pharmacopsychiatry 21:416–417, 1988

Schlegel S, von Bardeleben U, Wiedemann K, et al: Computerized brain tomography measures compared with spontaneous and suppressed plasma cortisol levels in major depression. Psychoneuroendocrinology 14:209–216, 1989a

Schlegel S, Maier W, Philipp M, et al: CT in depression: associations between ventricular size and psychopathology. Psychiatry Res 29:221–230, 1989b

Scott ML, Golden CJ, Ruedrich SL, et al: Ventricular enlargement in major depression. Psychiatry Res 8:91–93, 1983

Shima S, Shikano T, Kitamura T, et al: Depression and ventricular enlargement. Acta Psychiatr Scand 70:275–277, 1984

Spitzer RL, Gibson M, Endicott J: Global Assessment Scale. New York, New York State Department of Mental Hygiene, 1973

Spitzer RL, Endicott J, Robins E: Research Diagnostic Criteria for a Selected Group of Functional Disorders, 3rd Edition. New York, New York State Psychiatric Institute, 1978

Standish-Barry HMAS, Bouras M, Bridges PK, et al: Pneumo-encephalographic and computerized axial tomography scan changes in affective disorders. Br J Psychiatry 141:614–617, 1986

Sweeny D, Nelson C, Bowers M, et al: Delusional versus nondelusional depression: neurochemical differences. Lancet 2:100–101, 1978

Synek V, Reuben JR: The VBR using planimetric measurements of EMI scans. Br J Radiol 49:233–237, 1976

Tanaka Y, Hazama H, Fukuhara T, et al: Computerized tomography of the brain in manic-depressive patients: a controlled study. Folia Psychiatrica et Neurologica Japonica 36:137–144, 1982

Targum, SD, Rosen LN, DeLisi LE, et al: Cerebral ventricular size in major depressive disorder: association with delusional symptoms. Biol Psychiatry 18:329–336, 1983

Taylor MA, Redfield J, Adams R: Neurophysiological dysfunction in schizophrenia and affective disease. Biol Psychiatry 16:467–478, 1981

Wechsler D: Wechsler Adult Intelligence Scale-Revised. San Antonio, TX, Psychological Corporation, 1981

Weinberger DR, DeLisi LE, Perman GP, et al: Computed tomography in schizophreniform disorder and other acute psychiatric disorders. Arch Gen Psychiatry 39:778–783, 1982

Wilson RS, Fox JH, Huckman MS, et al: Computed tomography in dementia. Neurology 32:1054–1057, 1982

World Health Organization: International Classification of Diseases, 9th Revision. Geneva, World Health Organization, 1977

Zatz LM, Jernigan TL: The ventricular brain ratio on computed tomography scans: validity and proper use. Psychiatry Res 8:207–214, 1983

Chapter 2

Magnetic Resonance Imaging in Primary Affective Disorder

Peter Hauser, M.D.

Magnetic resonance imaging (MRI) is a technique that is based on the phenomenon of nuclear magnetic resonance (NMR) and involves an amalgamation of magnetic and radio transmitter technology. Its development rests on the theory and hardware of image processing and image reconstruction originating in the computer sciences. In psychiatry and neurology, MRI is predominantly utilized to study brain structure and to identify areas of tissue pathology. MRI can also be used to quantify ventricular and extraventricular intracranial cerebrospinal fluid (CSF) volumes and CSF flow. Potential applications exist for the in vivo analysis of hydrogen- and phosphorus-containing metabolites in the brain by nuclear magnetic spectroscopy and for measurement of cerebral blood flow and metabolism with paramagnetic tracers.

A comparison of computed tomography (CT) and MRI scans through the transverse plane highlights the differences between the two techniques (Figure 2-1). As can be seen, MRI allows excellent gray and white matter resolution of cortical and subcortical areas. The head of the caudate and other basal ganglia are clearly visualized with distinct margins that permit relatively easy measurement.

MRI allows scanning in the sagittal and coronal planes and therefore is not limited to the transverse plane as is CT. Imaging in the sagittal plane permits visualization of the corpus callosum and other midline structures (Figure 2-2a). Also, cortical bone, because of the short T2 relaxation time, has little signal to the image. Therefore, bone is essentially invisible. The posterior fossa, and the temporal

I wish to acknowledge the following colleagues who assisted in various aspects of this work: L. Altschuler, W. Berrettini, I.D. Dauphinais, T. Huggins, A. Rosoff, and R.M. Post. Particular thanks to A.J. Dwyer and M.V. Seeman for their editorial comments and C. Meyer for her help in creating the illustrations.

lobes, hippocampus, cerebellum, and brain stem, normally obscured by bone artifact on CT, are easily visualized in the coronal plane (Figure 2-2b). Unlike CT, MRI is without radiation risk to the patient and thus lends itself to sequential studies. This is particularly important in the investigation of the affective disorders, because patients can be scanned in different mood states while on and off medications. MRI with contrast enhancement is a more sensitive imaging modality than CT in demonstrating virtually all brain pathology, including tumors (McGinnis et al. 1983; Smith et al. 1985) and plaques secondary to demyelinating diseases, such as multiple sclerosis (Jacobs et al. 1986; Runge et al. 1984). The superiority of MRI over CT in detecting brain tissue pathology, particularly in the temporal lobe, has been demonstrated in several studies of patients with temporal lobe epilepsy (Jabbari et al. 1986; Kuzniecky et al. 1987; Riela et al. 1984; Theodore et al. 1986). CT, however, remains superior for the demonstration of acute hemorrhage, intracerebral calcifications, and bone detail (Bradley 1986).

This chapter is organized into two sections and an appendix. In the first section, I discuss the application of MRI technology to the study of brain structure with a particular emphasis on methodological aspects. In the second section, I review the findings of MRI studies in the affective disorders at the National Institute of Mental Health and those of other investigators. The appendix is a brief review of the basic principles of NMR and MRI.

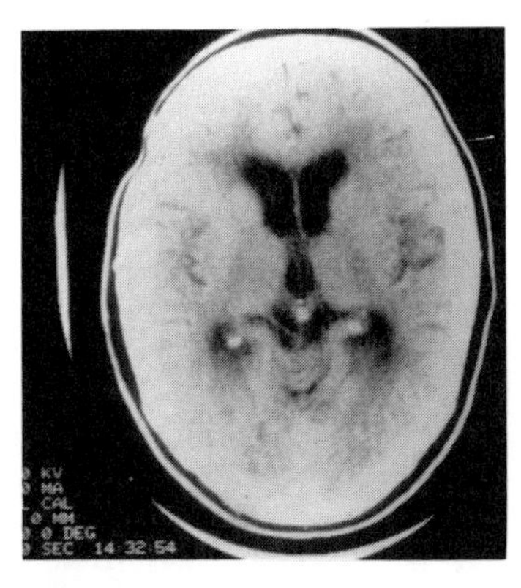

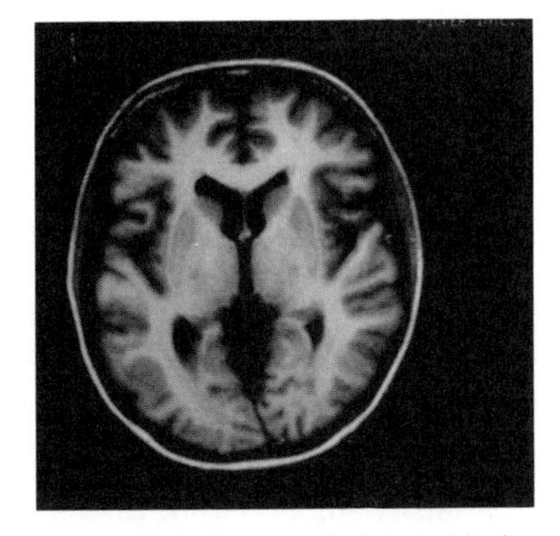

Figure 2-1. Comparison of CT and MRI. Transverse section through the basal ganglia (inversion recovery MRI, inversion time [TI] = 600 msec, repetition time [TR] = 3,250 msec, echo time [TE] = 30 msec.

APPLICATION OF MRI TECHNOLOGY: METHODOLOGICAL AND CLINICAL CONSIDERATIONS

The application of MRI to the study of the brain in psychiatric illnesses is still in its infancy, particularly with respect to the affective disorders. MRI technology in psychiatry was initially utilized to attempt to replicate CT scan studies that suggested structural abnormalities in illnesses such as schizophrenia. With time, however, it was realized that the superior resolution of MRI and its capacity to image in multiple planes provided unrestricted access to brain structures not visualized with CT. MRI thus permits a more specific and innovative investigational approach. Also, unlike CT, in which the relative density of structures is fixed and contrast directly reflects radiodensity, MRI provides a range of information as pulse sequences can be manipulated to enhance contrast between tissues or structures of interest. It is these complex possibilities that make MRI a potentially more powerful, but methodologically more demanding, tool than CT.

Methodological issues and clinical and demographic variables pertinent in imaging studies of brain morphology will be discussed. Particular attention is given to the study of patients with affective disorders.

Methodological Issues: MRI Technology

The vast majority of MRI studies of the brain have focused on examining structural abnormalities. There are essentially two types of structural studies: 1) T1 weighted pulse sequences (either inversion recovery or short spin-echo), which enhance contrast between normal structures and thus reflect anatomy; and 2) T2 weighted pulse sequences (long spin-echo), which enhance contrast between the normal and the abnormal, thereby revealing pathology. The selection of a particular pulse sequence is determined by the hypothesis to be investigated. The availability of different types of pulse sequences is important, as there exists great variation in MRI scanners and associated computer software available. For an explanation of pulse sequences, please see the appendix. Examples of T1 weighted and T2 weighted images are shown in Figure 2-3.

The selection of the imaging plane depends on the structure of interest; the midline sagittal section provides excellent visualization of such structures as the corpus callosum, cerebellum, and frontal and occipital lobes. The greatest amount of anatomic information is probably provided by coronal sections. The basal ganglia and limbic

A

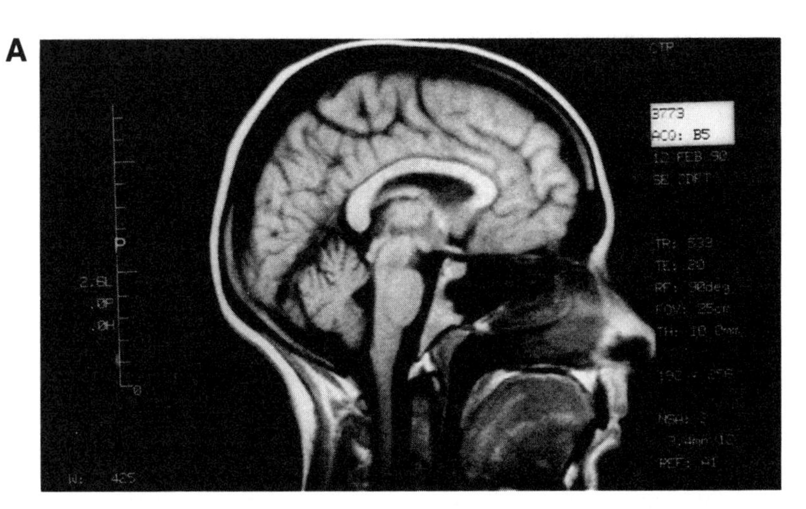

Figure 2-2. *A:* Midsagittal MRI scan (spin-echo MRI, repetition time [TR] = 533 msec, echo time [TE] = 20 msec). Corpus callosum, septum pellucidum, midbrain, and cerebellum are easily visualized. *B:* Sequential coronal sections, thickness 10 mm (inversion recovery MRI, inversion time [TI] = 600 msec, TR = 3,250 msec, TE = 30 msec). 10-mm thickness. First section is most posterior.

structures, including the hippocampus and amygdala, are easily visualized in this plane. Also, sequential coronal sections cut perpendicular to the frontal and temporal lobes and to the lateral ventricles allow delineation and volumetric quantification of these structures. Coronal sections are of particular utility in measuring the lateral ventricles; they provide a crisp boundary between ventricle and brain tissue, thus minimizing the problem of partial volume effect found in the measurement of transverse sections.

Standardization of head orientation in the scanner is of prime importance in brain imaging studies, as it is a potential source of error in subsequent measurement of structures. Early CT scan studies rarely controlled the angle of the transverse plane or the level of the initial slice, and this resulted in considerable variation of the image from subject to subject. Initial MRI studies at the National Institutes of Health (NIH) positioned the subject's head by laser light relative to the canthomeatal plane and obtained coronal sections perpendicular to this plane. Subjects often reposition their heads while in the scanner, however, which results in variability of the angle of coronal sections away from the perpendicular and leads to marked intersubject

B

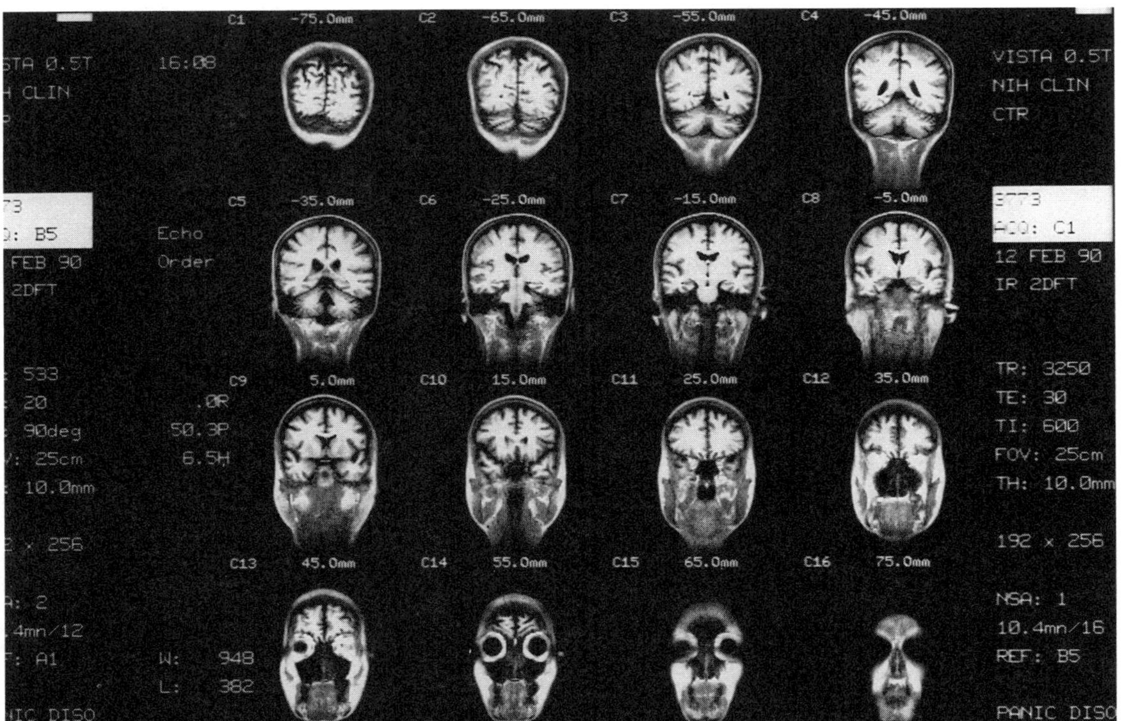
C1 -75.0mm
C2 -65.0mm
C3 -55.0mm
C4 -45.0mm
C5 -35.0mm
C6 -25.0mm
C7 -15.0mm
C8 -5.0mm
C9 5.0mm
C10 15.0mm
C11 25.0mm
C12 35.0mm
C13 45.0mm
C14 55.0mm
C15 65.0mm
C16 75.0mm
16:08
Echo
Order
.0R
50.3P
6.5H
W: 948
L: 382
VISTA 0.5T
NIH CLIN
CTR
12 FEB 90
IR 2DFT
TR: 3250
TE: 30
TI: 600
FOV: 25cm
TH: 10.0mm
192 x 256
NSA: 1
10.4mn/16
REF: B5

differences in the measurement of areas of interest. Subsequent studies have utilized oil-based capsules placed in the external auditory canal and at the corner of the eye (lateral canthus or angulus oculi lateralis) as markers of the canthomeatal line. T1 weighted sagittal sections are obtained, and the capsules appear as two small areas of hyperintensity on a lateral sagittal section (Figure 2-4a). The angle of the canthomeatal line relative to the horizontal plane is calculated, and a grid of the coronal sections perpendicular to the angle of the canthomeatal line is superimposed on the midsagittal section (Figure 2-4b). This technique permits a more reliable comparison of structures of interest among subjects. Also, the grid of the coronal sections can be consistently rotated a set number of degrees away from the perpendicular of the canthomeatal line. This allows coronal sections to be cut perpendicular to the longitudinal axis of structures of interest, which provides crisper margins for measurement. In an ongoing study of patients with affective disorder at NIH, a particular interest has been imaging the hippocampus. It was determined that coronal sections cut perpendicular to a longitudinal axis that is rotated 25° below the canthomeatal line provided optimal resolution of this structure (Figures 2-4d and e). The angle of coronal sections in this study is similar to an MRI study of hippocampal abnormalities in amnestic patients by Press et al. (1989), albeit the method of deter-

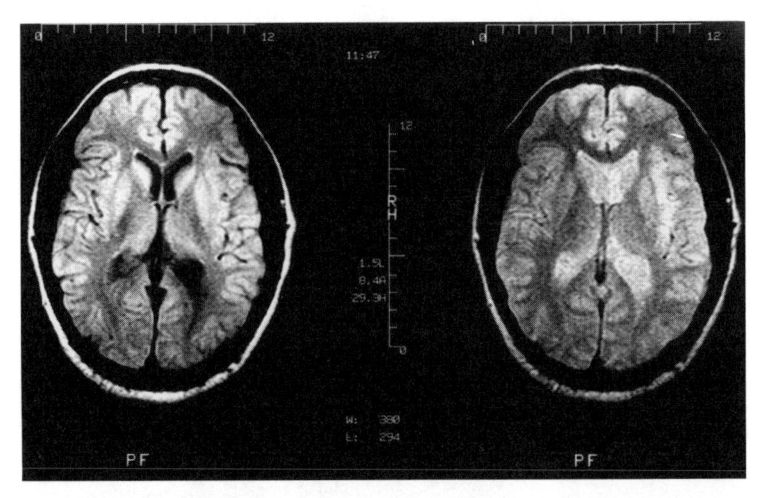

Figure 2-3. Comparison of T1 weighted (*left*) and T2 weighted (*right*) scans in the transverse plane. T1 weighted scan (spin-echo MRI, repetition time [TR] = 533 msec, echo time [TE] = 20 msec). T2 weighted scan (spin-echo MRI, TR = 2,000 msec, TE = 80 msec).

mining this angle and the width of the sections are both different. A coronal section perpendicular to the canthomeatal plane and cut at the same level as the section in Figure 2-4e is shown for comparison in Figure 2-4c.

Because there are variations in the size and shape of the brain, positioning of the coronal grid is important to ensure that structures of interest appear in the same section in different individuals. Selection of a central coronal section as a reference section minimizes the variability in measurement of structures in a series of coronal sections. Andreasen et al. (1990) selected the coronal section that cuts through the optic chiasm as a reference section. In studies of patients with affective disorders at NIH, the preference has been to utilize the coronal section that cuts through the pons as a reference section since the pons is a landmark that is easily identified in the midsagittal image and since this section cuts through the middle of the temporal lobes. The coronal grid is superimposed on the midsagittal image such that the anterior border of the pons is positioned in the midline of the section anterior to the central or reference section. The image produced has several distinct landmarks, including the pons, the peduncles, the interpeduncular cistern, and the third ventricle (Figure 2-4e).

Morphometric analyses of structures of interest vary greatly and are determined in large part by the weighting of the magnetic resonance image. As mentioned earlier, there are two types of structural studies undertaken in MRI of the brain: 1) T1 weighted scans, which enhance anatomic differences between normal structures such as gray and white matter or CSF and brain parenchyma and therefore are conducive to quantitative techniques of measurement; and 2) T2 weighted scans, which enhance differences between normal and abnormal or pathologic tissue and obscure differences in normal anatomy, and are perhaps best evaluated with qualitative methods (e.g., visual rating scales).

Quantitative techniques for measurement of structures visualized in T1 weighted images are not standardized, and new techniques such as three-dimensional volumetric reconstruction are still under development. Initial MRI studies utilized techniques and measured structures previously described in CT scan studies. These included linear and area measurements of the ventricular system. Area measurements continue to be the most popular means for assessing structures of interest and are made with either manual or computerized methods. Manual methods are often cumbersome and involve enlarging the hard copy image, tracing the outline of structures of interest, and measuring the areas with a hand-held planimeter. Various computerized methods for area measurement are in use; one method allows the

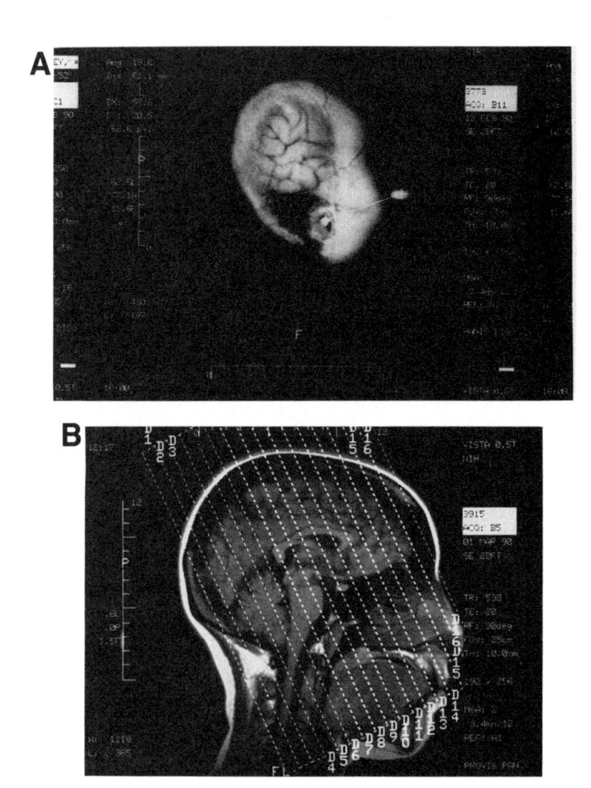

Figure 2-4. *A:* Head orientation relative to the canthomeatal plane. Oil-based capsules appear as bright objects on T1 weighted scans. In this figure, the capsules are placed in the external auditory canal and at the canthus and are marked with a cursor. The angle of the canthomeatal plane (*upper left*, Ang = 24.8) is calculated relative to the horizontal plane. (Scan: spin-echo, repetition time [TR] = 533 msec, echo time [TE] = 20 msec). *B:* Grid of the coronal sections perpendicular to the angle of the canthomeatal plane is superimposed on the midsagittal section (Scan: spin-echo, TR = 533 msec, TE = 20 msec). *C:* Resultant coronal section (corresponding to section D7 in *B*) when the grid is perpendicular to the canthomeatal plane. This coronal section does not cut perpendicular to the longitudinal axis of the hippocampus, and the boundary of the structure is not clearly demarcated. (Scan: inversion recovery MRI, TI = 600 msec, TR = 3,250 msec, TE = 30 msec). *D:* Grid of the coronal sections rotated 25° below the perpendicular to the angle of the canthomeatal plane (Scan: spin-echo, TR = 533 msec, TE = 20 msec). *E:* Resultant coronal section (corresponding to section C7 in *D*) when the grid is rotated 25° below the canthomeatal plane. This coronal section cuts perpendicular to the longitudinal axis of the hippocampus.

C

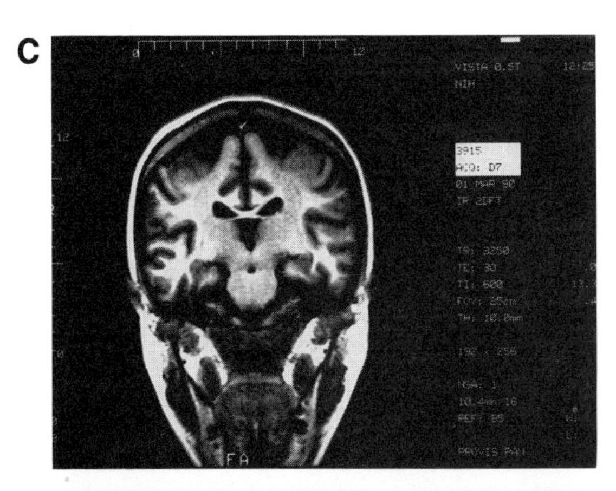
VISTA 0.5T
NIH
3915
ACQ: D7

D

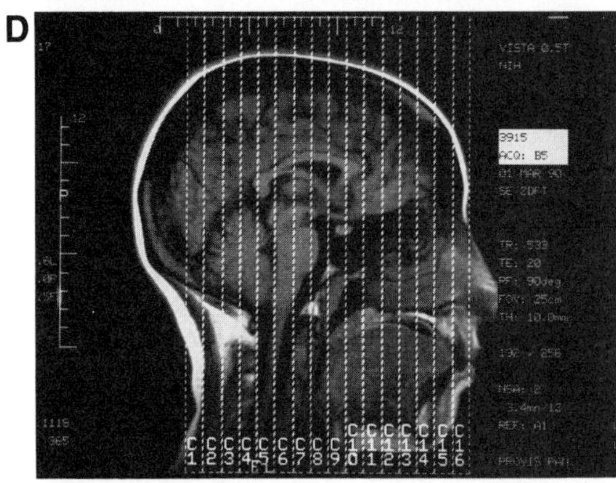
VISTA 0.5T
NIH
3915
ACQ: B5

E

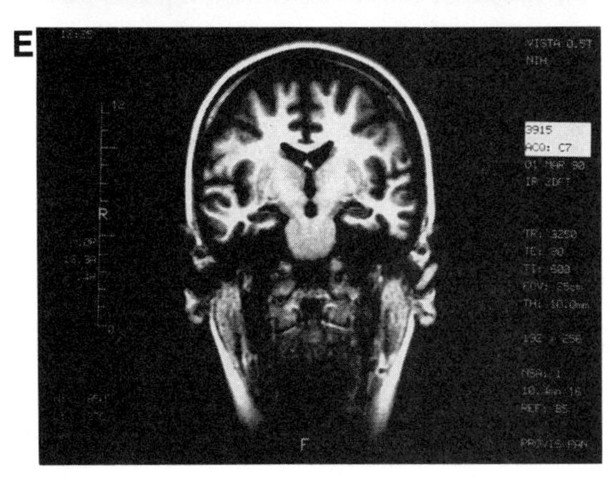
VISTA 0.5T
NIH
3915
ACQ: C7

rater to isolate a particular area of interest and then apply an automated edge detection technique to delineate the perimeter and calculate the area automatically. Computer programs, however, are unable to make judgments or distinguish between different structures that may have the same optical density. A more useful method is computer-assisted planimetry; the rater outlines the perimeter of a structure of interest by use of a cursor on an MRI computer console screen and then has the computer automatically calculate the area.

Volumetric measurements have been a more recent development in the quantitative analysis of brain structure. Initial studies summed area measurements on sequential coronal sections to obtain a volume estimate of such brain regions as the frontal and temporal lobes, the lateral ventricles, and the hippocampus. Although this method does provide information about the overall size of a particular structure or region, it is at best an estimate based on sequential two-dimensional samples of a three-dimensional volume that disregards the irregular boundaries of a particular structure. This technique is limited to large brain structures or regions because most scanners can only produce sections 5–10 mm thick. Small structures are not visualized in enough sections to provide an adequate estimate. Three-dimensional volume reconstruction based on images collected in multiple planes provides a more accurate estimate of the volume of a structure, but these computer programs are prohibitively expensive and still under development.

T2 weighted scans are utilized to assess the presence or absence of focal abnormalities, which appear as areas of hyperintensity. It has been postulated that these hyperintensities reflect a pathologic increase in tissue water resulting in a prolonged T2 relaxation time. Pathologic processes that cause hyperintensities include neoplasms, head trauma, multiple sclerosis, and atherosclerotic processes such as subcortical arteriosclerotic encephalopathy. In psychiatry, studies have focused on subcortical white matter hyperintensities in the periventricular and deep white matter regions and on hyperintensities in the subcortical gray matter nuclei, including the basal ganglia and thalamus. As these areas of hyperintensity are usually small or punctate, most studies simply note the presence and location of the lesion. A modification of a 4-point visual rating scale described by Fazekas et al. (1987) has been used to measure the severity of periventricular and deep white matter hyperintensities (Coffey, Chapter 4, this volume; Coffey et al. 1988b). Areas of hyperintensity have been noted in individuals with no evidence of psychiatric or neurologic illness. Therefore it is important not to ascribe pathologic significance to subtle differences that may be physiologic.

In summary, several methodological variables related to MRI technology contribute to disparity among MRI studies. As MRI scanners differ in the pulse sequences and computer software available, the selection of pulse sequences will vary from center to center and thus make comparison among studies difficult. Methods to control for differences in head orientation and head size can reduce variations in the images obtained from subject to subject and among studies. Consensus is urgently needed to standardize methods of measurement and thus to allow comparison among studies. Examples illustrating the existing variation in methods of measurement are the numerous MRI studies of the corpus callosum. This structure has been arbitrarily divided into either halves, thirds, fourths, or fifths without apparent regard to naturally occurring boundaries.

Methodological Issues: Clinical Variables

The affective disorders are a heterogeneous group of illnesses characterized by episodic alterations of mood. Clinical symptoms are diverse, and many different criteria are used to diagnose affective disorder. To make matters more complex, variations occur in the nutritional, neuroendocrinologic, and biochemical parameters of affective illness. These variations exist both among patients, and within the same patient, as a consequence of treatment or mood state.

It is the inherent heterogeneity of the affective disorders that makes the identification of relatively homogeneous subgroups difficult. This may explain, in part, the disparity of CT and MRI findings in the affective disorders. Despite these disparities, CT scan and postmortem neuroanatomic studies have provided important information on clinical and demographic variables that affect brain morphology. These variables as they pertain to MRI studies of patients with affective disorder will now be considered.

Cortisol status. The cortisol status of patients with an affective disorder is an important variable (see Schlegel, Chapter 1, this volume). Neuroendocrine hypotheses in affective disorder arose, in part, because of consistent observations that major depression is associated with alterations in hypothalamic functions subserving stress responsiveness, food intake, growth, and reproduction. Prominent among these observations are state-related abnormalities of the hypothalamic-pituitary-adrenal axis as reflected by elevations of plasma cortisol (Halbreich et al. 1984; Stokes et al. 1984), urinary free cortisol (Carroll et al. 1976; Stokes et al. 1984), and postdexamethasone cortisol levels (Brown et al. 1979; Carroll et al. 1981). Studies of affectively ill patients have reported a correlation of both elevated levels of urinary free cortisol excretion (Kellner et al. 1983) and elevated plasma cortisol levels (Schlegel et al. 1989) to larger ventricular brain ratios (VBRs). This suggests the possibility that endogenous steroids can alter the size and appearance of brain structures in the same way that exogenous steroids do (Bentson et al. 1978; Momose et al. 1971). As cortisol abnormalities are found in some but not all patients with affective disorder, the relationship of this variable to structural brain abnormalities is important to assess.

Although the interaction of cortisol and temporal lobe structures such as the hippocampus have not yet been studied in humans, studies in preclinical models raise interesting considerations. Animal studies have indicated that prolonged glucocorticoid exposure, induced either exogenously or by stress, reduces hippocampal neuronal number and produces changes similar to that found in the aged hippocampus (Sapolsky et al. 1985). Also, glucocorticoid elevation enhances hippocampal neuronal vulnerability to such insults as kainic acid (Sapolsky 1986) and ischemia (Sapolsky and Pulsinelli 1985). The potential relevance of these findings to the human is speculative, but the relationship of specific abnormalities of temporal lobe structures including the hippocampus to cortisol status and to cognitive deficits is ascertainable by MRI studies in the affective disorders.

Symptom picture. The symptom picture may also be related to variations in brain morphology among affectively ill patients. Episodes of illness are often characterized by a profound increase or decrease in weight. Decreased body weight has been reported to correlate with decreased brain size in postmortem studies (Ho et al. 1980b; Skullerud 1985). An extreme example are the CT scan studies of anorexia nervosa that show cortical atrophy and ventricular enlargement partially reversible after weight gain and normalization of endocrine and metabolic abnormalities (Krieg et al. 1988).

CT scan studies comparing affective patients with and without psychotic symptoms have reported greater changes of the ventricular system in patients with psychosis (Schlegel and Kretzschmar 1987). Whether the psychotic symptoms are antecedent to or a consequence of ventricular abnormalities is unknown.

Comparison of patients with unipolar versus bipolar illness or endogenous versus nonendogenous depression have not found robust differences in ventricular measurements between groups. Also, most studies have not found a relationship between the VBR and the duration of illness, number of episodes, or number of hospitalizations. However, one follow-up CT scan study of affectively ill patients that compared the VBR of initial and second CT scans (mean 35.2 months after initial scan) found a significant increase in the VBR over time (Vita et al. 1988). This suggests a progressive alteration of cerebral structures, the origin of which is unknown.

Mood state. The mood state is another parameter of affective illness that may vary within a given sample of patients. Postdexamethasone cortisol, urinary free cortisol, and plasma cortisol levels that are elevated during the acute phase of the illness usually normalize as the patient returns to a state of euthymia. Similarly, nutritional status and weight return to baseline. If structural abnormalities are a consequence of state-related changes, uniformity in the mood state of the patient sample is of importance.

The effect of medications. Different medications may produce changes on MRI as a result of fluctuations in water content of brain tissue. Drug doses may also be relevant. Rangel-Guerra et al. (1983) reported an increased T1 relaxation time in the frontal and temporal lobes of bipolar patients in the depressed phase. This decreased to that of normal controls after 10 days of lithium treatment. However, the normal controls in this study showed no changes in T1 relaxation time after treatment with similar doses of lithium. This suggests that specific changes in the behavior of water may play a role in bipolar disorder and in the therapeutic effect of lithium. In an NMR study of the red blood cells of six bipolar depressed patients, Rosenthal et al. (1986) reported significantly higher T1 relaxation times than in controls. After 1 week of lithium therapy, the T1 relaxation times significantly decreased in five of six patients. The decrease was associated with a clinical response to lithium. A more recent study found no differences in T1 relaxation time of brain regions between bipolar patients and controls (Besson et al. 1987), but patients were scanned after long-term treatment with lithium. Lithium's effect on intracellular or extracellular water content of the brain could manifest as structural changes. The effect of antidepressants on T1 or T2 relaxation times has not been studied.

In summary, the inherent heterogeneity of affective illness presents a difficult challenge while simultaneously offering a potential opportunity for imaging studies of the brain. Consideration of the various clinical parameters of affective illness may improve the homogeneity of the patient sample studied. As MRI is without radiation risk, it is a valuable tool that allows the same patient to be scanned in the acute and remitted phase of illness or on and off medication, thus permitting investigation of structural abnormalities as state or trait findings. This will ultimately improve our understanding of the pathophysiologic mechanisms that underlie the structural brain abnormalities observed in the affective disorders.

Methodological Issues: Demographic Variables

Neuroanatomic studies of the brain, evaluated by postmortem, CT, and MRI techniques, have described variations in quantitative brain indices and in brain structures in relationship to certain demographic variables.

Age. Age may contribute to variations in brain size. Postmortem studies have reported a decrease in brain weight with increasing age (Ho et al. 1980a; Skullerud 1985). Also, although there is controversy over the question of whether cortisol secretion increases with age in normal subjects, several studies of patients with affective disorder have observed a correlation of basal and postdexamethasone cortisol levels with age (Halbreich et al. 1984; Nelson et al. 1984; Stangle et al. 1986; Stokes et al. 1984; Weiner et al. 1987).

An increased prevalence of white matter hyperintensities on MRI scans has been reported in demented and nondemented elderly subjects (Rezek et al. 1987). The presence of these abnormalities has been shown to be associated with the increased systolic blood pressure that accompanies old age (Inzitari et al. 1987).

Sex-related differences. Sex-related differences exist not only in postmortem brain weight (Ho et al. 1980a; Skullerud 1985) but also in cerebral area as measured on midsagittal MRI scans (Hauser et al. 1989a). Postmortem studies suggest that women have smaller brains than men even when the difference in body length is taken into account (Skullerud 1985), but that the rates of decrease in brain weights as a function of age are significantly slower in women than in men (Ho et al. 1980a).

Sex-related differences have been reported in postmortem studies of the size and shape of the corpus callosum (De Lacoste-Utamsing and Holloway 1982; Holloway and De Lacoste-Utamsing 1986). However, these findings have not been replicated in other postmortem studies (Bell and Variend 1985; Demeter et al. 1988; Weber and Weis 1986; Witelson 1985) or in MRI studies (Bleier et al. 1986; Kertesz et al. 1987; Oppenheim et al. 1987), although the differences in techniques of measurement among studies do not permit adequate comparison.

Another sex-related consideration is the hormonal fluctuation that takes place during the menstrual cycle. One MRI study that scanned nonpsychiatrically ill women at midcycle and again premenstrually found relative increases in total cranial and lateral ventricular CSF volume premenstrually (Grant et al. 1988). The CSF volumes did not fluctuate appreciably on repeat measurement either in men or in postmenopausal women. Again, it is uncertain whether such changes would be reflected in quantitative neuroanatomic studies.

Laterality-related differences. Laterality-related differences may also be a source of variation in quantitative brain imaging studies as functional differences between the hemispheres may translate into neuroanatomic asymmetry. Postmortem studies have described right-left differences in the planum temporale and the Sylvian fissure (Galaburda et al. 1979; Geschwind and Levitsky 1968; Wada et al. 1975). The planum temporale is usually larger on the left in left-hemisphere–dominant individuals, which is thought to reflect greater development of the left hemisphere for language-related tasks. MRI studies have reported that the right temporal lobe volume is larger than the left in normal subjects (Jack et al. 1988; Suddath et al. 1989). Similar findings have been reported in temporal lobe volume measurements of schizophrenic patients (Suddath et al. 1989) and measurement of temporal to cerebral area ratios of affective patients (Hauser et al. 1989b). Also, CT (Chui and Damasio 1980; LeMay and Kido 1978) and MRI (Suddath et al. 1989) studies have reported that the right frontal lobe is larger than the left in normal subjects.

Callosal size has been reported in postmortem studies to be increased in left-handed and ambidextrous subjects compared to right-handed individuals (Witelson 1985, 1989). However, this finding has not been replicated in MRI studies of the corpus callosum (Bleier et al. 1986; Kertesz et al. 1987). Differences in the method of measurement make comparison of studies difficult. There seems to be a great variation in the size and shape of the corpus callosum regardless of hand preference or sex. The functional significance of this is not known.

Educational level. Educational level has recently gained attention as a possibly important variable to consider in structural imaging studies. In an MRI study that compared schizophrenic patients and normal controls, Andreasen et al. (1986) reported relatively decreased cranial, cerebral, and frontal lobe absolute areas (measured on the midsagittal section) in schizophrenic patients. However, a second study using the same techniques of measurement failed to replicate these findings (Andreasen et al. 1990). The discrepancy in the two studies appeared to be due to differences between the two groups of normal controls: the controls in study 1 had a significantly larger frontal lobe area and a trend toward a larger cerebral area than controls in study 2. The only demographic variable that differentiated the two groups of normal controls was educational level: in study 1 nearly all controls were college graduates, and many had received doctoral and postdoctoral training, whereas in study 2 controls were selected to more closely match the educational level of schizophrenic subjects and therefore had only a high school education or 1 to 2 years of college. The authors cautiously suggested that educationally advantaged individuals may achieve a complexity of cerebral organization that is reflected in an increased size of certain brain regions.

Selection of controls. The selection of normal controls is an important issue in structural brain imaging studies, particularly with respect to the affective disorders, because the differences observed between affective patients and controls have not been as robust as differences noted between schizophrenic patients and controls. One study of 121 subjects who presented themselves as normal, healthy volunteers and underwent structured interviews with the Schedule for Affective Disorders and Schizophrenia (Endicott and Spitzer 1978) disclosed that 16.5% of subjects met Research Diagnostic Criteria (RDC) (Spitzer et al. 1978) for diagnoses of current mental disorder and that, of the remaining subjects without current psychopathology, 35.6% had a past history of mental illness (Halbreich et al. 1989). Of the illnesses represented, the majority were affective disorders and alcoholism. If there are indeed state- or trait-related changes of brain structure in the affective disorders, inclusion of subjects with a current or past history of psychiatric illness as normal controls will serve to blur differences between subjects and normal controls.

In summary, it is of the utmost importance to compare affectively ill patients to demographically similar nonill controls who have no history of psychiatric or neurologic illness or substance abuse. If there are state- or trait-related changes of brain structure in the affective disorders, then using as normal controls individuals with a current or past history of psychiatric illness will obscure any specific brain changes that may be present. Also, data analysis should include examination of the effect and interaction of demographic variables such as age, sex, and laterality on the dimensions of structures of interest.

MRI STUDIES IN THE AFFECTIVE DISORDERS

As already mentioned, the majority of MRI studies undertaken in the affective disorders have investigated brain structure and can be divided into two types: 1) T1 weighted scan studies, which quantitate the area and volume of structures and regions of the brain; and 2) T2 weighted scan studies, which utilize visual analogue scales to assess the severity of pathologic abnormalities in the periventricular and basal ganglia regions. Although several additional MRI studies of affectively ill patients have been presented at conferences, the majority of studies reviewed in this section are those available at the time of writing in the published literature.

T1 Weighted Studies

There have been few quantitative MRI studies of patients with affective disorder. The brain regions examined by MRI in affective patients have been the same ones already identified as potentially interesting in studies of schizophrenia. They include the VBR, temporal lobes and limbic structures, the corpus callosum, and the frontal lobes.

VBR studies. In an MRI study of 10 patients with affective disorder (7 bipolar, 3 unipolar) and 10 normal subjects, no statistically significant differences were found in the VBR or T1 times between patient and control groups (Besson et al. 1987). All of the patients were euthymic and on therapeutic blood levels of lithium at time of scan. The controls were significantly younger than the patients, but the sex distributions of the two groups were the same. Height and weight of the patients and subjects were not reported.

A subsequent MRI study examined the relationship of the VBR to postdexamethasone cortisol levels and to the presence of white matter hyperintensities in 46 patients who satisfied DSM-III (American Psychiatric Association 1980) criteria for a diagnosis of major depression (Rao et al. 1989). The mood state and medication were not reported. A strong correlation was found between the highest postdexamethasone cortisol level and the VBR ($r = .51$, $P = .0003$). This correlation remained significant after age was factored out of the analysis (partial $r = .43$, $P = .003$). Nonsuppressors as a group had a significantly higher VBR than suppressors. No information was included on the severity of depression for each patient. In addition, patients with white matter hyperintensities had a greater VBR than those without such hyperintensities, but were significantly older. No controls were scanned in this study; therefore the relationship of white matter hyperintensities to an increased VBR is not necessarily attributable to affective illness. It may be a consequence of the aging process.

Temporal and frontal lobe studies. In a preliminary MRI study of 17 patients with affective disorder (mean age, 40.5 years) and 21 normal controls (mean age, 33.8 years), a coronal section through the temporal lobes at the level of the pons (Figure 2-4e) was selected in each subject, and the area of specific temporal lobe structures and the cerebrum were measured (Hauser et al. 1989b). All but two patients met RDC for bipolar affective disorder; the two remaining patients were unipolar depressed. Almost all patients were in a euthymic state and on medications (predominantly lithium) at the time of the scan. The control group was only informally screened for psychiatric or neurologic illness, had significantly more years of education, and was younger than the group of affectively ill patients. Structures of interest, including the hippocampal complex (hippocampus and parahippocampal white), white and gray matter of the temporal lobes, and the cerebrum, were traced on a blind basis for the right and left hemispheres and computed with the VAX/VMS computer system. Ratios between structures of interest were used to control for certain demographic variables, such as the height, weight, age, and sex of the subjects. No differences were found between affective patients and controls in the ratios of hippocampal complex to temporal lobe or cerebrum areas, and the ratio of the white to gray matter area of the temporal lobes. However, the temporal lobe to cerebrum area ratio was significantly smaller in patients than controls on the left ($t = -2.47$, 36 df, $P < .02$) and on the right ($t = -2.56$, 31/2 df, $P < .03$). As affective patients were significantly older than controls, the temporal lobe to cerebrum area ratio was reanalyzed after removing 5 patients over the age of 50; the remaining 12 patients had the same mean age (33.8 years; range, 18–48 years) as controls (range, 23–45 years). The temporal lobe to cerebrum area ratio remained significantly smaller in the left ($t = -2.15$, 31 df, $P < .04$), but was only at a trend in the right ($t = 1.81$, 30/7 df, $P < .08$) hemisphere. The relationship of certain clinical variables, including a history of psychosis, age of onset, and duration of illness, to the temporal lobe to cerebrum area ratio was examined. No correlation of the ratio to history of psychosis or age of onset was found. However, the temporal lobe to cerebrum area ratio was inversely correlated to duration of illness in the right hemisphere only ($r = -.49$, $P < .05$). Cerebral laterality differences were also noted; the temporal lobe to cerebrum area ratio was significantly smaller in the left than right hemisphere in both the affective and control groups (paired *t*-test: affective group, $t = 4.17$, 16 df, $P < 0.0007$; controls, $t = -4.76$, 20 df, $P < .001$). The right temporal lobe to left temporal lobe area ratio was greater than 1.0 in 13 of 17 affective patients and in 17 of 21 control subjects. None of the left-handers ($n = 5$) had a reversal of this asymmetry.

In a preliminary MRI study of 30 elderly (>60 years of age) depressed patients and 23 normal elderly controls with similar age, height, sex, and socioeconomic status, the volumes of particular brain regions were calculated from contiguous 5-mm coronal sections (Coffey et al. 1989a). The mood state and medication were not reported. All the subjects were right handed, and none had a history of neurologic illness. Elderly depressed patients had significantly greater total lateral ventricular volume (31.8 ml versus 21.7 ml, $P<.03$) and significantly smaller total frontal lobe volume (222.9 ml versus 250.5 ml, $P<.007$) than normal control subjects. No significant differences were noted in the total volumes of the cerebral hemispheres, temporal lobe, amygdala-hippocampal region, posterior hemispheres, or third ventricle between the two groups.

Another MRI study of 30 young bipolar patients (mean age, 33 years) and 52 normal controls (mean age, 28.8 years) measured various brain regions on the midsagittal section and assessed cognitive functioning with a comprehensive neuropsychological battery (Nasrallah et al. 1988). The mood state and medication were not reported. Comparison of the two groups revealed a high degree of cognitive impairment in bipolar patients and a significant correlation of poorer cognitive performance with smaller frontal and cerebral area measurements in both bipolar and normal control groups.

Corpus callosum studies. An MRI study of 24 schizophrenic patients, 22 bipolar patients, and 25 normal controls without medical or psychiatric history resulted in relative measurements of specific callosal dimensions and the cerebral area on the midsagittal section (Hauser et al. 1989a). The technique of measurement employed has been described in a previous study of schizophrenic patients (Nasrallah et al. 1986) and is shown in Figure 2-5. All of the bipolar patients met RDC and DSM-III criteria for bipolar disorder, were on some psychotropic medication (predominantly lithium), and were considered euthymic at the time of scanning. Age, sex, number of left-handers, and height did not differentiate the affective patients from the normal control subjects. No significant differences were found among diagnostic groups in anterior, mid, or posterior callosal width, callosal area, cerebral area, callosal to cerebral area ratio, or the genu (first quartile) to splenium (fourth quartile) ratio. The corpus callosal length was shorter in affective subjects than controls ($t = 3.04$, 44 df, $P<.04$). Significantly, sex differences were found in the corpus callosal and cerebral areas and in the genu to splenium ratio. Two-way analysis of variance showed a main effect for sex, indicating that men had a larger corpus callosal area ($F = 5.55$, 1/65 df, $P<.02$), a larger cerebral area ($F = 10.26$, 1/65 df, $P<.002$), and a smaller genu to splenium ratio ($F = 5.61$, 1/65 df, $P<.02$) than women.

T2 Weighted Studies

The T2 weighted MRI studies of young and elderly patients with affective disorder have described subcortical hyperintensities in the periventricular white matter and in the basal ganglia and have suggested an association between these abnormalities and certain clinical

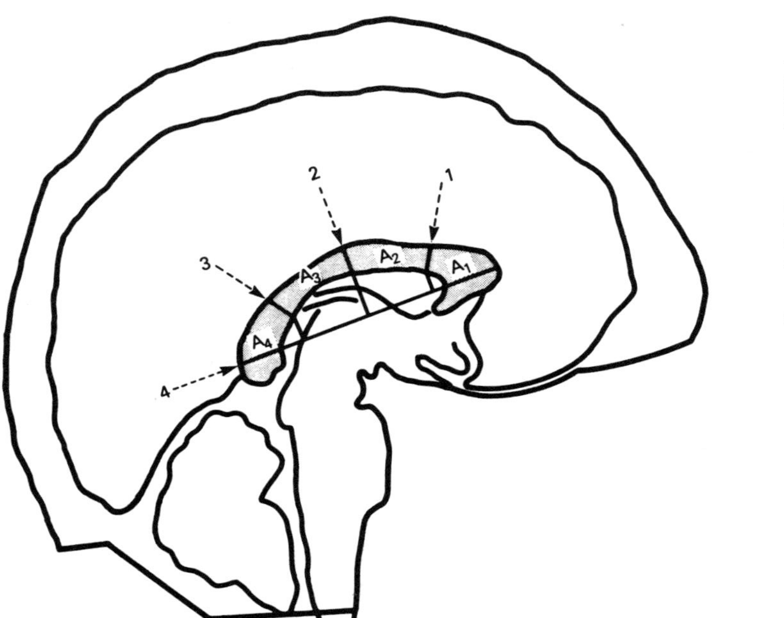

Figure 2-5. The technique of measurement. The maximum anterior-posterior callosal length (*4*) was divided into four quarters, and at the three points dividing the callosal length into four quarters, perpendiculars were extended to intersect with the ventral callosal wall. At the three intersection points with the ventral wall, perpendiculars to the ventral wall were drawn, dividing the corpus callosum into quartiles. The anterior callosal width (*1*) is the boundary between A_1 and A_2. The midcallosal width (*2*) is the boundary between A_2 and A_3. The posterior callosal width (*3*) is the boundary between A_3 and A_4. Reproduced with permission from Hauser et al. (1989a).

variables. However, similar changes have been noted on MRI scans of elderly normal subjects without neurologic illness, and differences between affective patients and normal controls may be in the severity or degree of these changes rather than in their occurrence.

In a study of 14 relatively young bipolar patients and 8 normal controls, subcortical hyperintensities were noted in 8 of 14 patients and in none of the controls (Dupont et al. 1987). The presence of these abnormalities was associated with a greater number of hospitalizations, but no significant differences were found between patients with and patients without hyperintensities in age, family history of affective illness, education, age of onset, history of psychosis, or medication use. A subsequent study of 19 bipolar patients and 10 age-matched controls, which included an unreported number of patients and normal subjects from the initial MRI study, again found subcortical hyperintensities only in the affectively ill group. These subcortical abnormalities were associated with greater impairment on cognitive tests of fluency and recall. Seven of nine patients with abnormalities were rescanned 1 year after the initial study. No patient showed either resolution or worsening of the subcortical hyperintensities, although four of these patients were in clinically different mood states from that of the initial MRI study.

Another MRI study assessed the presence or absence of subcortical hyperintensities in 35 inpatients who met criteria for major depression (Krishnan et al. 1988). The patients were divided into two groups: 12 below the age of 45 and 23 above the age of 45. There were no normal controls. In the group below age 45, 3 patients exhibited hyperintensities; 14 of the patients over age 45 had similar changes. Among the patients over age 45, subcortical abnormalities were more common in patients with a first episode of depression after age 45 than in patients who developed their first episode of depression prior to age 45. In a subsequent study of 46 patients who satisfied DSM-III criteria for a diagnosis of major depression, subcortical hyperintensities were found in 15 patients (Rao et al. 1989). The patients with white matter hyperintensities had a greater VBR than those without such hyperintensities, but were significantly older. No controls were scanned in this study; therefore, the relationship of white matter hyperintensities to an increased VBR is not necessarily attributable to affective illness, but may be a consequence of the aging process.

In a series of case reports and retrospective clinical studies on elderly depressed patients referred for electroconvulsive therapy, structural abnormalities, including subcortical hyperintensities, were found in two-thirds of patients examined (Coffey et al. 1987, 1988a, 1988b; Figiel et al. 1989). More than half of these patients had their first depressive episode after the age of 60. A more recent prospective MRI study of the elderly depressed and normal elderly controls, which utilized visual analogue scales to rate the severity of periventricular and deep white matter hyperintensities, reported subcortical white matter hyperintensities in all 51 patients scanned and at least moderately severe changes in half the patients (Coffey et al. 1989b). Of these patients, 80% had their first depressive episode after age 60. A second prospective MRI study of elderly depressed patients and normal elderly controls found that although periventricular and deep white matter hyperintensities were found in both groups, abnormalities were more common and more severe in the patient group (Coffey et al. 1990). These MRI studies and their clinical implications are discussed in greater detail by Coffey (Chapter 4, this volume).

CONCLUSION

MRI represents a new generation of scanning technology that provides anatomic and pathologic information superior to that obtained by CT. T1 weighted magnetic resonance images offer excellent gray-white matter resolution and improved visualization of brain tissue in the sagittal and coronal as well as transverse planes without bone artifact. This is of value in examining the posterior fossa, temporal lobes, cerebellum, and brain stem (regions obscured by bone artifact on CT images). Midline structures are also well visualized. T2 weighted magnetic resonance images permit the detection of pathologic lesions, particularly lesions in the white matter and basal ganglia secondary to tumors, cerebrovascular phenomena such as small infarctions, or demyelinating diseases such as multiple sclerosis.

Clinically, MRI is a useful diagnostic screening procedure that enables the clinician to detect the presence of a neuropathologic process that manifests as a psychiatric illness. However, as MRI scans are more expensive than CT scans, they are less often performed as the first study when brain pathology is suspected.

MRI is a powerful research method to study brain structure in the affective disorders, a method not yet utilized to its full potential. The initial MRI studies of patients with affective illness have examined the hypotheses of previous CT scan studies or attempted to replicate the structural studies undertaken in schizophrenia. Although quantitative structural studies have suggested a smaller temporal to cerebral area ratio in relatively young euthymic and medicated bipolar patients (Hauser et al. 1989b) and smaller total frontal lobe volumes in elderly depressed patients (Coffey et al. 1989a) when compared to normal controls, the findings of the various structural studies, taken together, are inconsistent. Any conclusions that can be made at present are speculative at best. The variety of methods of measurement employed, the imaging plane and pulse sequence selected, and the lack of attention given to critical clinical and demographic variables preclude adequate comparisons among studies.

The T2 weighted studies of relatively young bipolar patients (Dupont et al. 1990) and elderly depressed patients (Coffey et al. 1989a, 1990) that have described hyperintensities in the periventricular white matter and in the basal ganglia have been more rigorous in their attention given to clinical and demographic variables. Although the subcortical hyperintensities described in a subgroup of young bipolar patients were not found in age-matched controls, a recent MRI study of patients with panic disorder reported white matter hyperintensities and other focal abnormalities, albeit predominantly in the temporal lobes (Fontaine et al. 1990). In studies of the elderly depressed, subcortical hyperintensities were frequently found in both patients and in normal controls, although the severity of these lesions was greater in the elderly depressed group. However, subcortical hyperintensities have also been described in demented patients, and their presence is strongly correlated with vascular disease and hypertension. The significance of these white matter hyperintensities is controversial, and further studies are necessary to elucidate the nature of these changes and their specificity to a particular illness. Studies that examine the relationship between subcortical hyperintensities and quantitative structural brain changes are also necessary.

In summary, consensus among investigators on the methods of measurement employed and on critical clinical and demographic variables is essential. Consideration of these issues will allow for greater homogeneity of the patient sample and more reliable comparability among studies.

Since MRI is a young technology, investigators have not yet realized its full potential. Alone among scanning techniques, MRI can track patients over time. As MRI is without radiation risk, multiple repeat studies can be undertaken in the same patient. This is of particular importance in the study of the affective disorders, as the patient shifts mood, improves, starts and stops treatment, or relapses. MRI allows assessment of brain morphologic changes that accompany neuroendocrine, biochemical, and physiologic alterations in these various conditions. Also, the effect of pharmacologic treatment on the brain can be examined by scanning patients on various doses of different medications. Finally, genetic factors that may contribute to structural brain abnormalities in the affective disorders can be assessed by scanning affected and unaffected family members of index subjects.

It is hoped that this chapter will contribute to the design of future studies that will fully utilize the potential of MRI technology and help elucidate the association between structural brain changes and neuroendocrine, neurochemical, and genetic trait markers in the affective disorders.

REFERENCES

American Psychiatric Association: Diagnostic and Statistical Manual of Mental Disorders, 3rd Edition. Washington, DC, American Psychiatric Association, 1980

Andreasen NC, Nasrallah HA, Dunn V, et al: Structural abnormalities in the frontal system in schizophrenia: a magnetic resonance imaging study. Arch Gen Psychiatry 43:136–144, 1986

Andreasen NC, Ehrhardt JC, Swayze VW, et al: Magnetic resonance imaging of the brain in schizophrenia: the pathological significance of structural abnormalities. Arch Gen Psychiatry 47:35–44, 1990

Bell AD, Variend S: Failure to demonstrate sexual dimorphism of the corpus callosum in childhood. J Anat 143:143–147, 1985

Bentson JR, Reza M, Winter J, et al: Steroids and apparent cerebral atrophy on CT scans. J Comput Assist Tomogr 2:16–23, 1978

Besson JA, Henderson JA, Foreman I, et al: An NMR study of lithium responding manic depressive patients. Magn Reson Imaging 5:273–277, 1987

Bleier R, Houston L, Byne W: Can the corpus callosum predict gender, age, handedness, or cognitive differences. Trends in Neuroscience 9:391–394, 1986

Bradley WG: Magnetic resonance imaging in the central nervous system: comparison with computed tomography, in Magnetic Resonance Annual, 1986. Edited by Kressel HY. New York, Raven, 1986, pp 8–122

Brown WA, Johnston R, Mayfield D, et al: The 24-hour dexamethasone suppression test in a clinical setting: relationship to diagnosis, symptoms, and response to treatment. Am J Psychiatry 136:543–547, 1979

Carroll BJ, Curtis GC, Davies BM, et al: Urinary-free cortisol excretion in depression. Journal of Psychological Medicine 6:43–50, 1976

Carroll BJ, Feinberg M, Greden JD, et al: A specific laboratory test for the diagnosis of melancholia: standardization, validation and clinical utility. Arch Gen Psychiatry 38:15–22, 1981

Chui HD, Damasio AR: Human cerebral asymmetries evaluated by computerized tomography. J Neurol Neurosurg Psychiatry 43:873–878, 1980

Coffey CE, Hinkle PE, Weiner RD, et al: Electroconvulsive therapy of depression in patients with white matter hyperintensity. Biol Psychiatry 22:626–629, 1987

Coffey CE, Figiel GS, Djang WT, et al: Effects of ECT upon brain structure: a pilot prospective magnetic resonance imaging study. Am J Psychiatry 145:701–706, 1988a

Coffey CE, Figiel GS, Djang WT, et al: Leukoencephalopathy in elderly depressed patients referred for ECT. Biol Psychiatry 24:143–161, 1988b

Coffey CE, Holt P, Weiner RD, et al: Quantitative brain magnetic resonance imaging in the depressed elderly. Poster presented at the annual meeting of the American College of Neuropsychopharmacology, Hawaii, December 10–15, 1989a

Coffey CE, Figiel GS, Djang WT, et al: Subcortical white matter hyperintensity on magnetic resonance imaging: clinical and neuroanatomic correlates in the depressed elderly. Journal of Neuropsychiatry 1:135–144, 1989b

Coffey CE, Figiel GS, Djang WT, et al: Subcortical hyperintensity on magnetic resonance imaging: a comparison of normal and depressed elderly subjects. Am J Psychiatry 147:187–189, 1990

De Lacoste-Utamsing C, Holloway RL: Sexual dimorphism in the human corpus callosum. Science 216:1431–1433, 1982

Demeter S, Ringo JL, Doty RW: Morphometric analysis of the human corpus callosum and anterior commissure. Human Neurobiology 6:219–226, 1988

Dupont RM, Jernigan TL, Gillin JC, et al: Subcortical signal hyperintensities in bipolar patients detected by MRI. Psychiatry Res 21:357–358, 1987

Dupont RM, Jernigan TL, Butters N, et al: Subcortical abnormalities detected in bipolar affective disorder using magnetic resonance imaging. Arch Gen Psychiatry 47:55–59, 1990

Endicott J, Spitzer RL: A diagnostic interview: the Schedule for Affective Disorders and Schizophrenia. Arch Gen Psychiatry 35:837–844, 1978

Fazekas F, Chawluk JB, Alavi A, et al: MR signal abnormalities at 1.5 T in Alzheimer's dementia and normal aging. American Journal of Neuroradiology 8:416–421, 1987

Figiel GS, Coffey CE, Weiner RD, et al: Brain magnetic resonance imaging in elderly depressed patients receiving electroconvulsive therapy. Convulsive Therapy 5:26–34, 1989

Fontaine R, Breton G, Dery R, et al: Temporal lobe abnormalities in panic disorder: an MRI study. Biol Psychiatry 27:304–310, 1990

Galaburda A, LeMay M, Kemper T, et al: Right-left asymmetries in the brain. Science 199:852–856, 1979

Geschwind N, Levitsky W: Human brain: left-right asymmetries in temporal speech. Science 161:186–187, 1968

Grant R, Condon B, Lawrence A, et al: Is cranial CSF volume under hormonal influence? an MR study. J Comput Assist Tomogr 12:36–39, 1988

Halbreich U, Asnis FM, Zumoff B, et al: Effect of age and sex on cortisol secretion in depressives and normals. Psychiatry Res 13:221–229, 1984

Halbreich U, Bakhai Y, Bacon KB, et al: The normalcy of self-proclaimed 'normal volunteers'. Am J Psychiatry 146:1052–1055, 1989

Hauser P, Dauphinais ID, Berrettini W, et al: Corpus callosum dimensions measured by magnetic resonance imaging in bipolar affective disorder and schizophrenia. Biol Psychiatry 26:659–668, 1989a

Hauser P, Altshuler LL, Berrettini W, et al: Temporal lobe measurement in primary affective disorder by magnetic resonance imaging. Journal of Neuropsychiatry and the Clinical Neurosciences 1:128–134, 1989b

Ho KC, Roessmann U, Straumfjord JV, et al: Analysis of brain weight, I: adult brain weight in relation to sex, race, and age. Arch Pathol Lab Med 104:635–639, 1980a

Ho KC, Roessmann U, Straumfjord JV, et al: Analysis of brain weight, II: adult brain weight in relation to body height, weight, and surface area. Arch Pathol Lab Med 104:640–645, 1980b

Holloway RL, De Lacoste-Utamsing MC: Sexual dimorphism in the human corpus callosum. Human Neurobiology 5:87–91, 1986

Inzitari D, Diaz F, Fox A, et al: Vascular risk factors and leucoaraiosis. Arch Neurol 44:42–47, 1987

Jabbari B, Gunderson CH, Wippold F, et al: Magnetic resonance imaging in complex partial epilepsy. Arch Neurol 43:869–872, 1986

Jack CR, Gehring DG, Sharbrough FW, et al: Temporal lobe volume measurement from MR images: accuracy and left-right asymmetry in normal persons. J Comput Assist Tomogr 12:21–29, 1988

Jacobs L, Kinkel WR, Polachini I, et al: Correlations of nuclear magnetic resonance imaging, computed tomography, and clinical profiles in multiple sclerosis. Neurology 36:27–34, 1986

Kellner CH, Rubinow DR, Gold PW, et al: Relationship of cortisol hypersecretion to brain CT scan alterations in depressed patients. Psychiatry Res 8:191–197, 1983

Kertesz A, Polk M, Howell T, et al: Cerebral dominance, sex and callosal size in MRI. Neurology 37:1385–1388, 1987

Krieg JC, Pirke KM, Lauer C, et al: Endocrine, metabolic, and cranial computed tomographic findings in anorexia nervosa. Biol Psychiatry 23:377–387, 1988

Krishnan KR, Goli V, Ellinwood EH, et al: Leucoencephalopathy in patients diagnosed as major depressives. Biol Psychiatry 23:519–522, 1988

Kuzniecky R, de la Sayette V, Ethier R, et al: Magnetic resonance imaging in temporal lobe epilepsy: pathologic correlations. Ann Neurol 22:341–347, 1987

Le May M, Kido DK: Asymmetries of cerebral hemispheres on computed tomograms. J Comput Assist Tomogr 2:471–476, 1978

McGinnis BD, Brady TJ, New PJ, et al: Nuclear magnetic resonance (NMR) imaging of tumors in the posterior fossa. J Comput Assist Tomogr 7:575–584, 1983

Momose KJ, Kiellberg RN, Kliman B: High incidence of cortical atrophy of the cerebral and cerebellar hemispheres in Cushing's disease. Radiology 99:341–348, 1971

Nasrallah HA, Andreasen NA, Coffman JA, et al: A controlled magnetic resonance imaging study of corpus callosum thickness in schizophrenia. Biol Psychiatry 21:274–282, 1986

Nasrallah HA, Coffman JA, Burnstein BA, et al: Cognitive deficits and MRI findings in bipolar disorder compared to controls. Paper presented at the annual meeting of the American College of Neuropsychopharmacology, San Juan, Puerto Rico, December 11–18, 1988

Nelson WH, Khan A, Orr WW, et al: The dexamethasone suppression test: interaction of diagnosis, sex and age in psychiatric inpatients. Biol Psychiatry 19:1293–1304, 1984

Oppenheim JS, Lee BCP, Nass R, et al: No sex-related differences in human corpus callosum size based on magnetic resonance imagery. Ann Neurol 21:604–606, 1987

Press GA, Amaral DG, Squire LR: Hippocampal abnormalities in amnestic patients revealed by high-resolution magnetic resonance imaging. Nature 341:54–57, 1989

Rangel-Guerra RA, Perez-Payan H, Minkoff L, et al: Nuclear magnetic resonance in bipolar affective disorders. American Journal of Neuroradiology 4:229–231, 1983

Rao VP, Krishnan RR, Goli V, et al: Neuroanatomical changes and hypothalamo-pituitary-adrenal axis abnormalities. Biol Psychiatry 26:729–732, 1989

Rezek DL, Morris JC, Fulling KH, et al: Periventricular white matter lucencies in senile dementia of the Alzheimer type and in normal aging. Neurology 37:1365–1368, 1987

Riela AV, Penry JK, Laster DW: Magnetic resonance imaging versus computerized cranial tomography in complex partial seizures (abstract). Epilepsia 25:650, 1984

Rosenthal J, Strauss A, Minkoff L, et al: Identifying lithium-responsive bipolar depressed patients using nuclear magnetic resonance. Am J Psychiatry 143:779–780, 1986

Runge VM, Price AC, Kirschner HS, et al: Magnetic resonance imaging of multiple sclerosis: a study of pulse-technique efficacy. American Journal of Neuroradiology 5:691–702, 1984

Sapolsky R: Glucocorticoid toxicity in the hippocampus: temporal aspects of synergy with kainic acid. Neuroendocrinology 43:440–444, 1986

Sapolsky R, Pulsinelli W: Glucocorticoids potentiate ischemic injury to neurons: therapeutic implications. Science 229:1397–1400, 1985

Sapolsky R, Krey L, McEwen B: Prolonged glucocorticoid exposure reduces hippocampal neuronal number: implications for aging. J Neurosci 5:1221–1226, 1985

Schlegel S, Kretzschmar K: Computed tomography in affective disorders, part I: ventricular and sulcal measurements. Biol Psychiatry 22:4–14, 1987

Schlegel S, von Bardeleben U, Wiedemann K, et al: Computerized brain tomography measures compared with spontaneous and suppressed plasma cortisol levels in major depression. Psychoneuroendocrinology 14:209–216, 1989

Skullerud K: Variations in the size of the human brain. Influence of age, sex, body length, body mass index, alcoholism, Alzheimer changes, and cerebral atherosclerosis. Acta Neurol Scand (Suppl) 102:1–94, 1985

Smith AS, Weinstein MA, Modic MT, et al: Magnetic resonance with marked T2-weighted images: improved demonstration of brain lesions, tumor, and edema. American Journal of Neuroradiology 6:691–697, 1985

Spitzer RL, Endicott J, Robins E: Research Diagnostic Criteria: rationale and reliability. Arch Gen Psychiatry 35:773–782, 1978

Stangle D, Pfol B, Zimmerman M, et al: The relationship between age and post-dexamethasone cortisol: a test of three hypotheses. J Affective Disord 11:185–197, 1986

Stokes PE, Stoll PM, Koslow SH, et al: Pretreatment DST and hypothalamic-pituitary-adrenocortical function in depressed patients and comparison groups. Arch Gen Psychiatry 41:257–267, 1984

Suddath RL, Casanova MF, Goldberg TE, et al: Temporal lobe pathology in schizophrenia: a quantitative magnetic resonance imaging study. Am J Psychiatry 146:464–472, 1989

Theodore WH, Dorwart R, Holmes M, et al: Neuroimaging in refractory partial seizures: comparison of PET, CT and MRI. Neurology 36:750–759, 1986

Vita A, Sacchetti E, Cazzullo CL: A CT scan follow-up study of cerebral ventricular size in schizophrenia and major affective disorder. Schizophrenia Research 1:165–166, 1988

Wada JA, Clarke R, Hamm A: Cerebral hemispheric asymmetry in humans. Arch Neurol 32:239–246, 1975

Weber G, Weis S: Morphometric analysis of the human corpus callosum fails to reveal sex-related differences. J Hirnforsch 27:237–240, 1986

Weiner MF, Davis BM, Mohs RC, et al: Influence of age and relative weight on cortisol suppression in normal subjects. Am J Psychiatry 144:646–649, 1987

Witelson SF: The brain connection: the corpus callosum is larger in left-handers. Science 229:665–667, 1985

Witelson SF: Hand and sex differences in the isthmus and genu of the human corpus callosum. Brain 112:799–835, 1989

Appendix

Basic Principles of MRI

MRI is based on the theory of NMR and the magnetic properties of the atomic nucleus. When the atomic nucleus of a chemical element contains an odd number of neutrons or protons, an intrinsic spin is produced, which generates a magnetic dipole oriented along the axis of spin. This acts like a miniature bar magnet associated with a magnetic field (Figure A-1). The strength and orientation of the dipole is called the magnetic moment. Magnetic moments can be conceptualized as vectors; that is, they have magnitude and direction. The sum of the magnetic moments or the vector sum of the individual protons is described as the net magnetization vector, M_O. MRI assesses this net magnetization vector.

The hydrogen nucleus, because it is simple (one proton only) and because it is abundant in the body, is the nucleus most commonly studied in MRI. Hence, clinical imaging is normally called proton imaging. In living tissue, the magnetic moments of the hydrogen atoms are oriented in random directions; thus the magnetic moments cancel one another out, resulting in a net magnetic moment of zero ($M_o = 0$). In the presence of a strong external magnetic field (B_o), the individual proton magnetic moments align with respect to the direction of the external field. This causes a net macroscopic magnetization of the tissue (Figure A-2).

In addition to aligning the hydrogen protons, the external magnetic field causes the spinning protons to precess about the z axis at

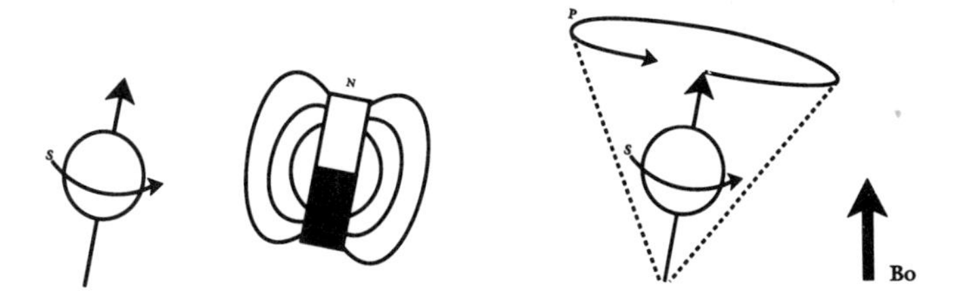

Figure A-1. Representation of a charged spinning proton. The intrinsic spin generates a magnetic dipole oriented along the axis of spin that acts like a bar magnet. S = spin, P = precession, B_o = external magnetic field. N = north.

a precessional or resonance frequency (ω_o) that depends on a constant specific for each nuclear species (the magnetogyric ratio γ), and the magnetic field strength (B_o). The Larmor equation expresses this relationship as: $\omega_o = \gamma B_o$.

EQUILIBRIUM

Magnetization is described in terms of an x-y-z coordinate system, with the z axis corresponding to the direction of the external magnetic field and perpendicular to the x-y plane. MRI is based on the assessment of the x-y component.

When placed in a magnetic field, the hydrogen protons eventually reach an equilibrium state in which the protons precess at the same frequency. Each of their vectors has the same z component but different x-y components. The individual x-y components cancel each other out and thus the net magnetization vector has a z component (M_z) but a zero x-y component (M_{xy}). This position of the net magnetization vector is called the equilibrium position (M_o) and is aligned along the z axis, corresponding to the direction of the external magnetic field (Figure A-3). At equilibrium, the net magnetization vector has no x-y component; therefore, there is no measurable signal.

EXCITATION

The signal assessed in MRI relates directly to the x-y component of the net magnetization vector. Since at equilibrium M_o has zero x-y

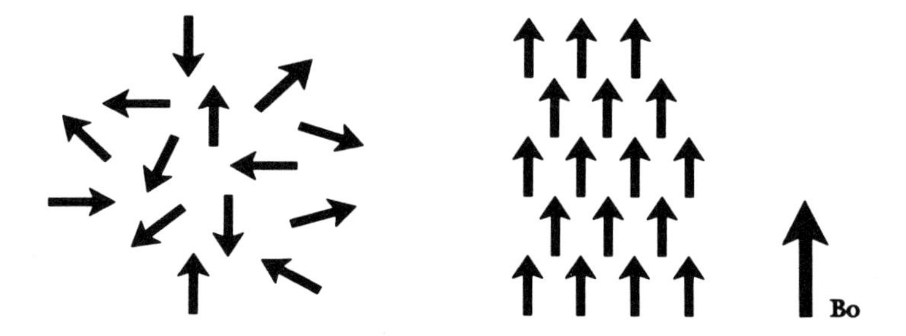

Figure A-2. The individual proton magnetic moments are represented as vectors. *Left:* In the absence of an external magnetic field, the magnetic moments are oriented in random directions and thus cancel one another out, resulting in a net magnetic moment of zero (M_o = net magnetic moment). *Right:* In the presence of an external magnetic field (B_o), the individual proton magnetic moments align with respect to the direction of the external magnetic field.

component, it must be displaced or rotated from the equilibrium position to produce a detectable signal. This is accomplished by an excitation pulse, which is a pulse of electromagnetic radiation at the same frequency as the precessing protons oriented along the x-y plane. During excitation, the protons acquire energy, and the net magnetization vector is rotated away from its equilibrium. The degree of rotation is dependent on the pulse's strength and duration. Pulses are named in terms of the degree of rotation they induce; a 90° pulse rotates M_O 90° from the z axis onto the x-y plane, a 180° pulse "inverts" M_O (i.e., rotates it from the positive to negative z axis).

As an example, during excitation with a 90° pulse, the net magnetization vector is deflected from the z axis onto the transverse or x-y plane (Figure A-3). The longitudinal or z component (M_z) is now zero and the x-y or transverse component (M_{xy}) is substantial.

RELAXATION

Relaxation is the transition of the net magnetization vector from the excited to the equilibrium state. Relaxation comprises two related processes: 1) the reconstitution of the longitudinal component (M_Z)—longitudinal or spin-lattice relaxation, and 2) the loss of the transverse component (M_{XY})—transverse or spin-spin relaxation. Longitudinal and transverse relaxation occur simultaneously and in an exponential fashion. The rapidity of longitudinal relaxation is determined by a time constant, T1, an exponential growth constant; the rapidity of transverse relaxation is determined by T2, an exponential decay constant.

T1, the longitudinal relaxation time, dictates the rate at which the longitudinal or z component (M_z) is reconstituted. T1 is defined as the time necessary for the z component (M_z) of the net magnetization vector to return to 63% of its equilibrium value. The longer the T1, the slower the z component returns to its equilibrium state. Longitudinal relaxation depends on the rate with which the energy of excitation is transmitted to the proton's surroundings (the lattice), hence the term *spin-lattice relaxation.*

T2, the transverse relaxation time, dictates the rate with which the x-y or transverse component (M_{xy}) is lost. T2 is defined as the time necessary for the x-y component (M_{xy}) of the net magnetization vector to decay to 37% of its excited value. The longer the T2, the slower the relaxation. Transverse relaxation is due to dephasing of the protons. Just after excitation, all protons are aligned and contribute completely to the net magnetization vector (M_{xy}). Over time, the individual protons dephase (Figure A-3), and, when completely dephased, the x-y component (M_{xy}) of the net magnetization vector is zero. As dephasing results from the interaction of hydrogen protons with one another, transverse relaxation is called spin-spin relaxation.

PULSE SEQUENCE

The signal intensity and therefore contrast is dependent on the NMR properties of the tissue (i.e., proton density, T1 relaxation time, and

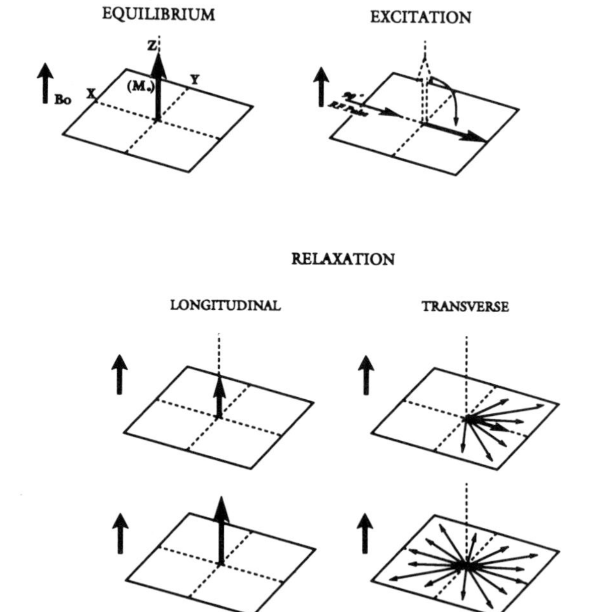

Figure A-3. Equilibrium: When placed in an external magnetic field, hydrogen protons reach an equilibrium in which the protons precess at the same frequency. The net magnetization vector has a z component (M_z) but a zero x-y component (M_{xy}). The position of the net magnetization vector is called the equilibrium position (M_o).
Excitation: Since at equilibrium M_o has zero x-y component, it must be rotated from the equilibrium position to produce a measurable signal with an excitation pulse. Pulses are named in terms of the degree of rotation they induce. In this figure, the radio frequency (RF) pulse is 90° as it rotates M_o 90° from the z axis onto the x-y plane.
Relaxation: The transition from the excited to the equilibrium state is called relaxation. Relaxation comprises two related processes: 1) the reconstitution of the longitudinal component (M_z)—longitudinal or spin-lattice relaxation—and 2) the loss of the transverse component (M_{xy})—transverse or spin-spin relaxation. Longitudinal and transverse relaxation occur simultaneously.

T2 relaxation time). The dependence of the signal on any one of these components is determined by the pulse sequence. A pulse sequence refers to a defined set of excitation pulses and interpulse spacing used to produce a discernible signal. By manipulating the pulse sequence, tissues of interest will show different signal intensities and produce maximum diagnostic contrast based on expected differences in T1 and T2 and proton densities. Two structures clearly distinguishable on one pulse sequence may be isointense on another. A pulse sequence that relies heavily on proton density is referred to as saturation recovery, but is infrequently used as it gives very poor contrast. More commonly used pulse sequences are influenced by either T1 or T2 relaxation times. The two types of pulse sequences in current use are spin-echo and inversion recovery.

Spin-echo pulse sequences, by varying the time between pulses, can be used to produce T1 weighted or T2 weighted images, although spin-echo is predominantly used to obtain T2 weighted images. This type of pulse sequence begins with a 90° excitation pulse followed by a short period of relaxation called echo time (TE), after which the signal is measured. A 180° inversion pulse is given halfway through TE to correct for the effects of inhomogeneity of the magnetic field. Following measurement there is a pause before a second 90° excitation pulse is given, and the cycle is begun again. The time between 90° excitation pulses is referred to as the repetition time (TR). By shortening the TE, T2 dependence is minimized, as the time allowed for transverse relaxation, the component determined by T2, is decreased. A long TE allows more time for transverse relaxation, thus accentuating differences in T2 and producing a T2 weighted image. TR defines the time allowed for longitudinal relaxation, the component determined by T1. A TR in the range of the T1 of the tissue of interest is optimal to produce T1 weighted images. A long TR allows for almost complete longitudinal relaxation and thus diminishes T1 weighting and accentuates T2. Spin-echo pulse sequences that produce T2 weighted images are less anatomically distinct, but more sensitive in detecting differences in tissue such as found in tumors or multiple sclerosis plaques.

Inversion recovery pulse sequences produce images with excellent gray-white matter resolution and are superior for visualization of anatomic structures. This type of pulse sequence begins with a 180° excitation pulse that inverts the net magnetization vector into the z axis. During relaxation, the net magnetization vector returns to its equilibrium value. However, as this relaxation occurs in the z axis, the x-y or transverse component of the net magnetization vector is zero and therefore not measurable. A second 90° pulse is necessary to deflect the net magnetization vector into the x-y plane in order for a measurable signal to be generated. The time between the 180° inversion pulse and the 90° pulse is called the inversion time (TI). After the 90° pulse and measurement is completed, another 180° inversion pulse is given, and the cycle is begun again. The time between 180° inversion pulses is referred to as TR. As T1 and T2 relaxation times are specific tissue characteristics, manipulation of the TI and TR allows for maximization of contrast between different tissues. Inversion recovery pulse sequences achieve great sensitivity to differences in T1 and therefore provide good anatomic display because of the disparity in T1 relaxation times among normal tissues. As this pulse sequence depends predominantly on T1 and contrast depends on differences in T1, the images are considered to be T1 weighted.

IMAGE RECONSTRUCTION

As the excited protons relax, they produce a signal that is recovered by a receiver coil. The signal measured reflects changes in the x-y component (M_{xy}) of the net magnetization vector. The signal comprises data collected about the amplitude and frequency of the signal emitted by the excited protons as the net magnetic vector returns to equilibrium.

The signal obtained from tissue placed in a static external magnetic field is an aggregate of signals generated from protons in different locations within the tissue and therefore contains no spatial information. To obtain an image, information on the location of the signal emitted from individual protons must be obtained. This is achieved by superimposing a linear magnetic field gradient on the static external magnetic field; gradient coils within the MRI scanner allow the signal to be localized and measured in slices of tissue, and series of slices can be reconstructed simultaneously. The signal emitted from individual protons will then depend on their position along the direction of the gradient field.

The signals measured by the receiver coil are analyzed into components arising from volume elements of tissue or voxels; these are transformed into an image by computer. In the image produced by MRI, the computer identifies the signal contribution of each voxel and reconstructs the voxel as a picture element or pixel. The level of gray assigned to each pixel is determined by the signal strength of its corresponding voxel. The image is composed of the numerous individual pixels and displayed as a black-and-white picture.

The signal intensity is dependent on the proton density, the T1 relaxation time, and the T2 relaxation time. The proton density is the number of protons in a given sample of tissue. T1 and T2 are explained above. Generally, an increased proton density, a decreased T1, and an increased T2 increase signal intensity and therefore brightness. However, the imaging sequences most commonly used are most influenced by either the T1 or T2 relaxation times. Tissues with a short T1 relaxation time return to equilibrium more rapidly and therefore have a greater signal intensity. Tissues with a long T2 relaxation time decay more slowly and also have a greater signal intensity.

Areas of the brain vary greatly in their T1 and T2 values. T1 is shortened as the molecular environment becomes more complex, due to the decreased mobility of hydrogen protons. White matter of the brain has a shorter T1 than gray matter, as hydrogen protons in water are bound in myelin sheaths surrounding axons and therefore appear bright on T1 weighted images. In comparison, cerebrospinal fluid has a longer T1 as does pathology that results in edema and thus appears dark on T1 weighted images. The rate of decay during T2 relaxation also differs among tissues. T2 is longer in white than gray matter of the brain and in pathologic processes, and longest in cerebrospinal fluid and water. The longer the T2 relaxation time, the brighter the tissue appears on T2 weighted images.

Examples of T1 weighted and T2 weighted images are shown in Figure 2-3.

Chapter 3

Positron-Emission Tomography and Mood Disorders

Barry H. Guze, M.D., Lewis R. Baxter, Jr., M.D., Martin P. Szuba, M.D., Jeffrey M. Schwartz, M.D.

Progress in mood disorders has been hampered by limits to the understanding of the underlying pathophysiology. Positron-emission tomography (PET) is unique in that it permits both visualization and quantification of cerebral biochemical processes. It is well tolerated and relatively noninvasive. However, because of the extensive work that must be done to develop a quantitative model for a specific biochemical process prior to the utilization of a new PET tracer, only a few biochemical processes have been studied to date. The majority of work with PET on mood disorders has been done with the glucose analogue fluorodeoxyglucose (FDG). Studies that measure blood flow and oxygen metabolism, amino acid pools, and serotonin receptor binding have also been performed.

Although the application of the PET technique to the study of mood disorders is in its infancy, it is an area where great progress toward understanding the pathophysiology of mood disorders can be expected.

FUNDAMENTAL PRINCIPLES OF PET SCANNING

PET is an analytical imaging technique that provides in vivo measurements of the anatomic distribution and rates of specific biochemical reactions (Phelps et al. 1979, 1985). It provides tomographic images and quantitative estimates of the distribution of compounds labeled with positron emitters (Phelps et al. 1983). Carbon, nitrogen, oxygen, and fluorine exist as short-lived isotopes that decay by positron emission (Table 3-1).

This work was supported in part by a contract (AM03-76-SF0012) from the U.S. Department of Energy, grant MH37916-02 and a Research Scientist Development Award (MH00752-02) (L.R.B.) from the National Institute of Mental Health, donations from the Jennifer Jones Simon Foundation, and the Judson Braun Chair in Psychiatry, University of California, Los Angeles.

Table 3-1. Half-lives of common positron-emitting isotopes

Nuclide	Half-life (min)
^{11}C	20.4
^{15}O	2.7
^{13}N	9.96
^{18}F	109.7

The emitted positron travels a few millimeters before combining with an electron. This results in the annihilation of the emitted positron by the electron. Two 511 KeV photons are produced and travel in opposite directions.

Detectors within the PET device, oriented at 180 degrees to each other, see these 511 KeV photons almost simultaneously. The circuitry of the PET device requires that the photons come from opposing directions within a time limit of about 5–20 nanoseconds to be counted. In addition, they must possess sufficient energy (usually 100–350 KeV) to activate the detectors. This process of recording photons is called coincidence detection (Figure 3-1).

Using a system of multiple detectors arranged in rings, these coincident events can be recorded with high efficiency. The nature of the PET device is such that it is able to recover a high percentage of the emitted activity and therefore is able to achieve a high-definition image that is a visual representation of the concentration of the positron-emitter-labeled chemical in a given anatomic region.

The technique of image reconstruction is a mathematical method known as "linear superimposition of filtered back projection." This is the superimposition of detected radiation, obtained from different angles, using appropriate mathematical processing to form tomographic images. It is the fundamental principle underlying all forms of computed tomography (CT). These filtered back-projection algorithms permit the reconstruction of a comprehensive set of radioactivity distribution images covering the whole brain. Current spatial resolution for PET is usually on the order of approximately 6 mm in all planes.

What these images represent depends on the physical and chemical properties of the radiolabeled tracer and on the mathematical model used to quantify the physiologic phenomena of interest. The concentration of radioactivity measured by PET can be converted into numerical estimates of the biochemical and physiologic processes governing the distribution of the labeled tracer. This process of quantification requires tracer kinetic models—mathematical representations of the distribution of the tracer and its quantification by

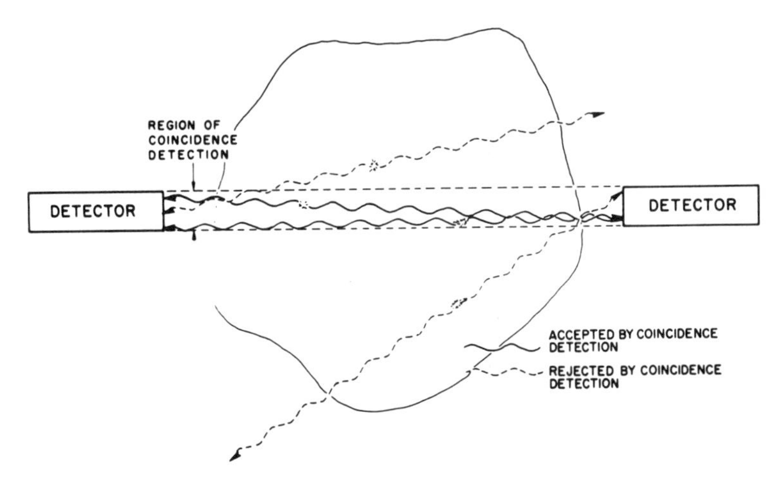

Figure 3-1. Schematic diagram of the principle of annihilation coincidence detection. When a positron comes into contact with an electron in the body, the two particles annihilate and produce two 511-KeV gamma rays that are emitted 180° to each other. If two gamma-ray detectors are placed on opposite sides of an object containing a positron emitter, the detection of two annihilation photons simultaneously, or in coincidence, places the original position of the annihilation in the space between the two detectors (between the *dashed lines*). Gamma rays from annihilations occurring outside this sensitive volume can interact with only one of the detectors per annihilation. By electronically selecting only those events seen in coincidence, all other events are rejected, and the coincidence events are localized to the region between the two detectors. Reprinted with permission from Phelps ME, Hoffman EJ, Mulani NA, et al: Application of annihilation coincidence detection to transaxial reconstruction tomography. J Nucl Med 16:210–224, 1975. Copyright 1975 Society of Nuclear Medicine.

the images. The FDG technique, which is utilized for the determination of local cerebral glucose metabolism in humans, is analogous to the 2-deoxyglucose autoradiographic method used in animals. FDG has unique properties. After intravenous injection, FDG enters the brain and is subsequently phosphorylated by brain hexokinase. The metabolic product, ^{18}F-labeled 2-deoxyglucose-6-phosphate (FDG-6-PO_4), remains trapped in neurons with only slow dephosphorylation. Unlike glucose, it is not metabolized further. This partly metabolized analogue of glucose allows assessment of brain metabolism over a brief interval while the image is recorded by the scanner. Since, along with oxygen, glucose is the predominant energy substrate for the brain, its metabolism reflects functional demand under normal conditions.

In a typical study, the patient receives an intravenous injection of FDG. For 30 minutes after the FDG is injected, blood sampling occurs. Blood is repetitively withdrawn in small samples for measurement of FDG and glucose. After approximately 30 minutes, between 85% and 95% of the neuronal uptake of FDG has occurred. FDG uptake is proportional to neuronal glucose metabolism. As part of the process of image quantification, the time course of ^{18}F activity and glucose concentration is determined by plasma measurement, while brain activity is determined by scanning. With the knowledge of predetermined rate constants, an operational equation allows calculation of local cerebral metabolic rate for glucose distributed on a cross-sectional picture (Huang et al. 1980; Phelps et al. 1979).

Because little FDG is converted or further metabolized during the next 40–120 minutes when image acquisition occurs, the metabolic rate signal remains stable during the first 30 minutes after FDG injection for acquisition by the scanner. Typically, two million counts per plane are required to achieve an adequate image. From these measurements, the images, composed of raw radioactivity counts, are converted into the actual glucose metabolic rate. This is usually expressed in micromoles or milligrams of glucose per 100 g of brain tissue per minute.

PET, MOOD, AND GLUCOSE METABOLISM: A REVIEW OF THE LITERATURE

Several studies have investigated glucose metabolism using PET (see Table 3-2).

Glucose metabolism was measured in 10 bipolar patients and 1 unipolar patient who met DSM-III (American Psychiatric Association 1980) criteria (Buchsbaum et al. 1984). All were depressed at the time of scanning and were drug free for at least 2 weeks. There were 19 normal control subjects. FDG was administered just before the subjects received a series of unpleasant 1-sec electrical stimuli to the right forearm for 34 minutes. Both normal subjects and patients showed an anterior to posterior gradient in absolute glucose use. The highest metabolic rates were in the occipital poles, but for normal subjects glucose use in preselected anterior cortical regions was greater than glucose use in selected posterior regions. A pattern of relative hypofrontality and relatively diminished anteroposterior gradients were also observed in patients with affective disorder. The authors concluded there is a relative hypofrontal function in bipolar depressive patients.

Using the PET-FDG technique, 24 patients with affective disorders and normal age-matched controls were examined (Baxter et al. 1985).

Table 3-2. PET scanning in mood disorders

Study	Diagnosis	Conditions	Resolution	Tracer	Findings
Buchsbaum et al. (1984)	10 bipolar depressed 19 controls	forearm shock eyes closed ears open	1.75 cm in plane 1.78 cm axial	FDG	Lower frontal:occipital metabolic ratios compared to controls (relative hypofrontality); relatively diminished anteroposterior gradients.
Baxter et al. (1985)	11 unipolar 5 bipolar depressed 5 mania 3 mixed-state 9 controls	eyes open ears open	11 mm in plane 12.5 mm axial	FDG	Bipolar depressed and mixed patients: low whole-brain metabolic rates. Rates increased as mood improved. Unipolar patients: low caudate/hemisphere ratio.
Buchsbaum et al. (1986)	16 bipolar depressed 4 unipolar 24 controls	eyes closed ears open forearm shock	1.75 cm in plane 1.78 cm axial	FDG	Bipolar patients: relative hypofrontality and low basal ganglia/hemisphere ratios versus controls. Unipolar patients: higher frontal/occipital ratios, relatively decreased basal ganglia metabolism.

Continued

Table 3-2. PET scanning in mood disorders (*continued*)

Study	Diagnosis	Conditions	Resolution	Tracer	Findings
Post et al. (1987)	5 moderate depression 7 mild depression 2 hypomanic 18 controls	eyes closed ears open forearm shock	1.75 cm in plane 1.78 cm axial	FDG	In moderate depression: maximum glucose use relative to maximums elsewhere in the same slice was significantly reduced in the right temporal lobe versus controls (trend on the left).
Baxter et al. (1989)	10 unipolar depressed 10 bipolar depressed 10 OCD with secondary depression 14 OCD without depression 12 controls	eyes open ears open	11 mm in plane 12.5 mm axial	FDG	Mean ratio of anterolateral prefrontal cortical metabolic rates to hemisphere rates low in depression versus controls. Left ALPFC lower in bipolar depressive than manic patients. Hamilton depression scores with left ALPFC metabolism. Successful drug treatment correlated with percentage of change in ALPFC.

Kishimoto et al. (1987)	9 unipolar depressed 3 manic 3 remitted depression 7 controls	eyes open ears open	11 mm in plane 12 mm axial	^{11}C-glucose	Lower ^{11}C-glucose in unipolar depression than in controls; bipolar metabolism higher than controls. ^{11}C-glucose activity correlates with amino acid pools.
Raichle et al. (1985)	4 unipolar depressed 1 bipolar depressed	not stated	not stated	^{15}O	Cerebral blood flow and cerebral metabolic rate for oxygen decreased versus controls. Cerebral blood volume not different from controls.
Mayberg et al. (1988)	8 left hemisphere strokes 9 right hemisphere strokes 17 controls	not stated	1.6 cm in plane	^{11}C-methyspiperone	Ratio of binding showed a negative correlation with severity of depression for left temporal cortex.

Note. FDG = fluorodeoxyglucose. OCD = obsessive-compulsive disorder. ALPFC = anterolateral prefrontal cortex.

There were 11 unipolar depressive patients, 5 bipolar depressive patients, 5 manic patients, and 3 mixed-state subjects, diagnosed using DSM-III criteria. Patients had moderate depression—21-item Hamilton Rating Scale for Depression (Hamilton 1967) score range, 17–25—and were drug free for at least 1 week before scanning. All bipolar patients had a documented prior manic episode observed by the patient's physician. Scans were performed in low ambient light with eyes and ears open. Subjects were not engaged in a specific task or stimulus condition. A NeuroECAT was used with in-plane resolution of 11 mm and axial resolution of 12.5 mm.

In this study whole-brain metabolic rates were significantly lower in bipolar depressed and bipolar mixed patients than in all other groups. The rates for bipolar depressed and mixed patients were similar. Whole-brain metabolic rates increased as patients' clinical state changed from bipolar depression to a euthymic or manic state. In the regional analyses, bipolar depressed patients had significantly lower metabolic rates for glucose in frontal, temporal, occipital, and parietal lobes, as well as the cingulate, caudate, and thalamus, in both hemispheres, when compared with unipolar depressed patients. Normal controls had a significantly higher glucose metabolic rate than the bipolar depressed group in frontal lobes, caudate, and thalamus.

Patients with unipolar depression showed a significantly lower ratio of the metabolic rate of the caudate nucleus divided by that of the hemisphere as a whole when compared to normal controls and patients with bipolar depression. The ratio of glucose metabolism in the caudate to that of the hemisphere for the unipolar depressed patients was significantly lower when compared with the normal controls and when compared with the bipolar depressed patients. When the five patients with unipolar depression were rescanned, the mean of this ratio increased for those patients who improved.

In the National Institute of Mental Health (NIMH) group (Buchsbaum et al. 1986), 16 patients with bipolar depression, 4 patients with unipolar depression, and 24 normal controls were studied with PET FDG. Many of these where the same patients reported in their other report. All had been free of psychoactive medication for a minimum of 14 days prior to study. All subjects underwent a semistructured interview based on the Schedule for Affective Disorders and Schizophrenia (Endicott and Spitzer 1978). Diagnoses were based on DSM-III criteria. All subjects were free of clinically significant abnormalities on physical examination or laboratory test. Control subjects were healthy according to history; neither they nor their first-degree relatives had a psychiatric history. Environmental conditions at the time of FDG uptake consisted of a dark room with the subjects' eyes closed and no conversation. Somatic sensory stimulation was administered to the right forearm during FDG injection. It consisted of a sequence of electrical stimuli ranging in intensity from barely perceptible to unpleasant.

Scanning was commenced approximately 35 minutes after injection and lasted 50–70 minutes. Seven or eight slices were obtained using an Ortec Ecat II (resolution 1.75 cm both in-plane and in the axial direction). A calculated attenuation correction was used for all studies.

Data were analyzed using several techniques. Three slices present in all individuals were used for cortical lateralization and determination of an anteroposterior gradient. The first slice was the supraventricular slice. It was the last slice down from the top where the gray central masses were not seen. It consisted mainly of cortical rim. The second slice was the midventricular slice containing the frontal cortex, insula, and Sylvian fissure. Mesial to that were the basal ganglia and the thalamus. The third slice was the infraventricular slice. This contained the lower frontal cortex, the tips of the temporal lobes, and parts of the cerebellum.

The first method of data analysis was the "cortical peel method." In this approach, the outer contour of each slice was outlined with a computer boundary-finding technique. This outlined area was divided to create a total of eight pie-shaped regions forming a frontal, midanterior, midposterior, and a posterior section on each side. Analysis of the outer rim of the brain slice (mainly cortex) was done by creating a 2.2-cm wide strip within and bordering the brain outline. Hypofrontality was a ratio of the anterior (frontal) to posterior sector of less than 1.0 and indicated a frontal metabolic rate less than the posterior metabolic rate. This ratio was calculated for the right and left sides separately and for the sum of the right and left sides. Bipolar patients had significantly lower frontal to occipital glucose metabolic ratios than normal controls. This has been termed a relative hypofrontality in bipolar illness. The ratio of the glucose metabolic rate in a sector to that of the whole slice showed bipolar patients to have lower ratios than normal controls in frontal cortex but no significant differences in occipital cortex. Thus relative hypofrontality in bipolar patients was attributable to relative frontal decreases rather than relative occipital increases.

The second method of data analysis was the region of interest method. An image from the brain atlas of Matsui and Hirano (1978) was used for reference. A 3 x 3 pixel box (about 0.3-cm cubed voxel) was placed in the center of each structure (caudate nucleus, putamen, anterior ventrolateral thalamus, median ventrolateral thalamus, posterior ventrolateral thalamus, superior frontal gyrus, globus pallidus, inferior putamen) by visual inspection. Mean glucose metabolic rates were calculated for the left and right side for each region. Analysis was carried out on both absolute values of glucose in micromoles per 100 g of tissue per minute and relative glucose use expressed as regions of interest divided by mean glucose metabolic rate in the whole slice. Patients with bipolar affective illness had significantly lower metabolic rates in their basal ganglia in comparison to whole slice metabolism than normal controls. Patients with unipolar depression showed relatively decreased metabolism in the basal ganglia. Clinical depression ratings correlated negatively with whole slice metabolic rate.

Mood disorder patients had metabolic rates higher than controls in the caudate and putamen regions for the lower slice. Rates were similar to control subjects for the caudate in the upper slice. Overall, average metabolic rates for all slices and structures were not significantly different. When expressed as a ratio to whole slice metabolic rate, both unipolar and bipolar patients had decreased glucose use in the basal ganglia as a whole and the caudate in particular compared to normal controls. This relative reduction was most striking in the right caudate.

The third technique for data analysis was the lateral cortical view method. The cortical peel was extracted from each slice. A line joining each successive pixel on a line to the center of the slice was calculated. All pixels in the peel transversed by this line were averaged. This averaging generated one mean cortical glucose value for each pixel in the slice outline. Lateral cortical surface analysis demonstrated a pattern of high glucose metabolism in the frontal cortex of normal subjects. This pattern was less marked in bipolar subjects.

The fourth method of data analysis was glucose consumption. Values of glucose use were calculated according to the Sokoloff (1977) model. Global metabolism was found to be significantly higher in subjects with affective illness (both unipolar and bipolar depressive) compared to normal controls.

In another study, glucose utilization in the temporal lobes of 13 patients with a history of mood disorders was compared with that of 18 normal volunteer controls (Post et al. 1987). These patients were part of the initial NIMH series, and some have, therefore, been reported before. The patients consisted of 5 depressed, 6 euthymic, and 2 manic individuals. The same individual was not studied as his or her mood states changed.

Maximum glucose use relative to any other maximums in the same PET image plane were calculated. In depressed patients, this relative measure was reduced on the right temporal lobe compared to normal volunteers. Temporal lobe glucose metabolism relative to other parts of the slice not only showed relative decreases in the depressed phase of the illness but progressive increases with improvement or euthymia and further increases in the two manic patients studied. There was no significant increase in glucose metabolism either as a maximum or in relation to other areas of the PET scan slice.

Regional cerebral glucose metabolism was examined in 10 patients with unipolar depression, 10 with bipolar depression, 6 with mania, 10 suffering from obsessive-compulsive disorder (OCD) with secondary depression, 14 afflicted with OCD without major depression, and 12 normal controls (Baxter et al. 1989). The depressed patient groups were matched for severity with the Hamilton Rating Scale for Depression. Subjects with OCD without depression and subjects with OCD with depression had similar levels of OCD pathology as determined by rating scales. Subjects were studied at rest with eyes and ears not occluded.

The middle frontal gyrus (dorsal anterolateral prefrontal cortex = ALPFC) was identified in all tomographic planes for each subject. The local glucose metabolic rate value was determined for each structure by weighing that structure's planar metabolic value by its cross-sectional area. This value was "normalized" by dividing it by the metabolic rate of the ipsilateral hemisphere.

The authors had hypothesized a priori that a cerebral dysfunction in the ALPFC would need to fulfill the following criteria to be considered a true state-dependent cerebral abnormality in depression.

1. The ALPFC/hemisphere ratio would be similar in both bipolar and unipolar depressions of equivalent severity, and signficantly different from that observed for normal controls and subjects with OCD but without major depression.
2. The ALPFC/hemisphere would distinguish OCD without depression from OCD with secondary major depression and, likewise, would distinguish bipolar mania from bipolar depression.
3. The degree of ALPFC/hemisphere deficit would correlate significantly with a standard measure of depression severity.
4. This ratio would change significantly in the direction of normal values in the same individuals on resolution of the depressed state.

The authors decided, again a priori, to examine the ALPFC/hemisphere because of previous 133 Xe blood-flow studies and other evidence implicating that region in depression. The left ALPFC/hemisphere satisfied all of these hypothesized criteria for a cerebral abnormality in depression, whereas the right ALPFC/hemisphere did not satisfy three of these criteria completely.

Mean glucose metabolic rates for the left ALPFC, divided by the rate for the ipsilateral hemisphere as a whole (ALPFC/hemisphere), were similar in the primary depressions (unipolar depression, bipolar depression) and were significantly lower than those in normal controls or those with OCD without depression (Figure 3-2). Results for the

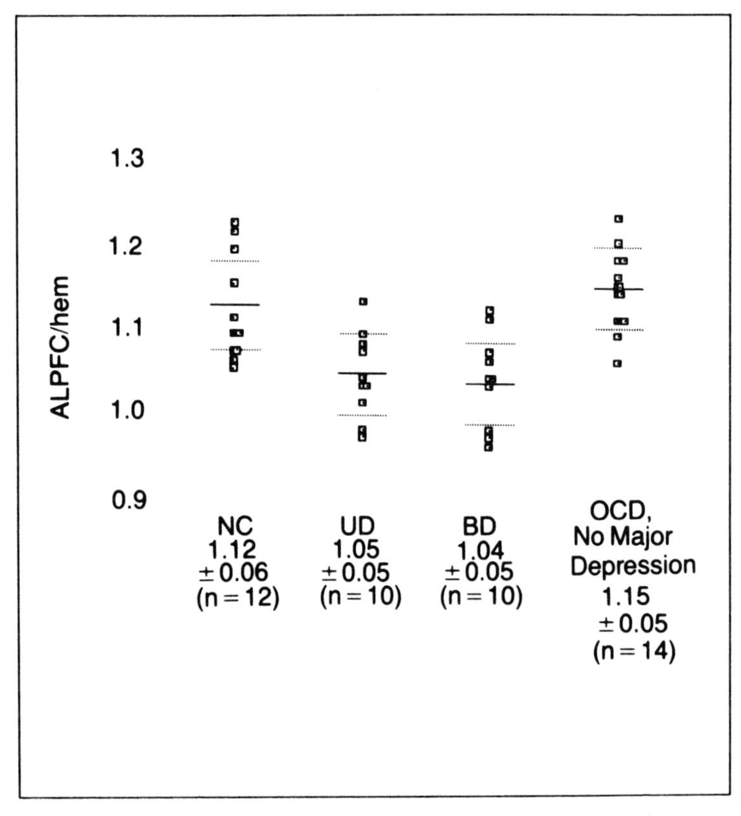

Figure 3-2. Mean (±SD) glucose metabolic rates for left middle frontal gyrus (dorsal anterolateral prefrontal cortex) divided by rate for entire hemisphere (ALPFC/hem). Ratio was significantly lower in patients with unipolar depression (UD) and bipolar depression (BD) than in either patients with obsessive-compulsive disorder (OCD) without secondary major depression or normal controls (NC) ($F = 12.74$, $P = 5 \times 10^{-6}$). Findings for right hemisphere were similar. Reprinted with permission from Baxter LR, Schwartz JM, Phelps ME, et al: Reduction of prefrontal cortex glucose metabolism common to three types of depression. Arch Gen Psychiatry 46:243–250, 1989. Copyright 1989 American Medical Association.

right hemisphere were similar for these comparisons. Values in subjects with OCD with depression were also significantly lower than in subjects with OCD without depression, but only on the left hemisphere (see Figure 3-3). Values in subjects with bipolar depression were lower than those in manic subjects on this measure in the left hemisphere, although results were not significant for the right hemisphere.

There was a significant negative correlation between the clinical depression severity scores (Hamilton Rating Scale for Depression) and the left ALPFC/hemisphere (Figure 3-4). With improvement of depression, the left ALPFC/hemisphere metabolic rate increased significantly, and the percent change in the Hamilton score correlated significantly with the percent change in the left ALPFC/hemisphere. For normal controls, and for bipolar depressive patients and unipolar depressive patients, the diagnostic groups on which the Hamilton was originally standardized, there was a significant negative correlation with the left and right ALPFC/hemisphere. Likewise, the Hamilton and the left ALPFC/hemisphere showed a significant negative correlation for a group combining patients with OCD with and without depression. There was not a significant correlation on the right.

Summary

The finding by Buchsbaum et al. (1986) of elevated global metabolism in patients with affective disorders contrasts with the report by Baxter et al. (1985), who found decreased global metabolism in depressed bipolar patients compared to normal controls or unipolar depressive patients. Baxter et al. found that the low global metabolism of the depressed state increased to normal levels in the euthymic state. Buchsbaum et al.'s negative correlation between metabolic rate and global depression ratings is in the same direction, however. One factor that may account for the differences in global metabolic findings was the psychological state or cognitive task that the subjects were engaged in at the time of FDG uptake. In unipolar depression, three studies not using the PET technique have found decreased global cerebral blood flow (CBF) (Gustafson et al. 1981; Mathew et al. 1980; Rush et al. 1982).

Bipolar and unipolar depressive patients could be differentiated by anteroposterior gradients of cortical glucose metabolism (Buchsbaum et al. 1986). Bipolar depressive patients had the lowest gradient; normal controls had an intermediate gradient, and unipolar depressive patients had the greatest gradient of the three groups. Baxter et al. (1985) found a greater decrease in frontal lobe glucose metabolism relative to normal controls in bipolar patients (40%) than they did for

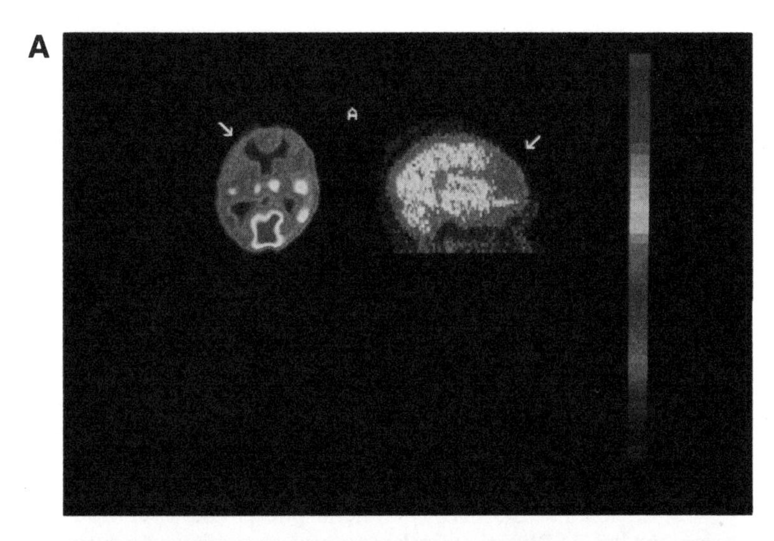

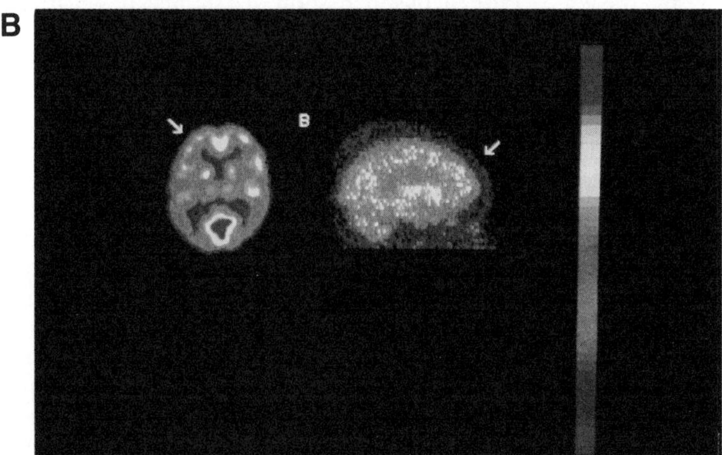

Figure 3-3. Positron-emission tomographic scans illustrating extreme case of low glucose metabolic rates in left dorsal anterolateral prefrontal cortex (*arrows*), divided by rate for hemisphere as a whole, in patient with severe obsessive-compulsive disorder with secondary major depression. Horizontal and rectilinear (lateral) views are shown. *A*: Disease state. *B*: Same patient 6 weeks later, after effective treatment with antidepressant medication. Reprinted with permission from Baxter LR, Schwartz JM, Phelps ME, et al: Reduction of prefrontal cortex glucose metabolism common to three types of depression. Arch Gen Psychiatry 46:243–250, 1989. Copyright 1989 American Medical Association.

parietal (28%) or occipital (29%) structures. In four unipolar depressive patients, Buchsbaum et al. found a larger anteroposterior gradient than found in normal controls or bipolar depressive patients. Baxter et al. (1989) found depressive patients had decreased lateral left prefrontal lobe metabolism. Different environmental conditions and stimuli during uptake may account for some of the difference in results.

Both bipolar and unipolar depressive patients had significantly lower relative caudate ratios compared to normal controls. The unipolar patients were lowest on the bottom two slices that contained these structures, whereas the bipolar patients were lowest on the top slice. The left-right difference (left greater than right) was largest for the bipolar group. Baxter et al. (1985) also found decreased relative ratios for caudate metabolic activity in unipolar depression.

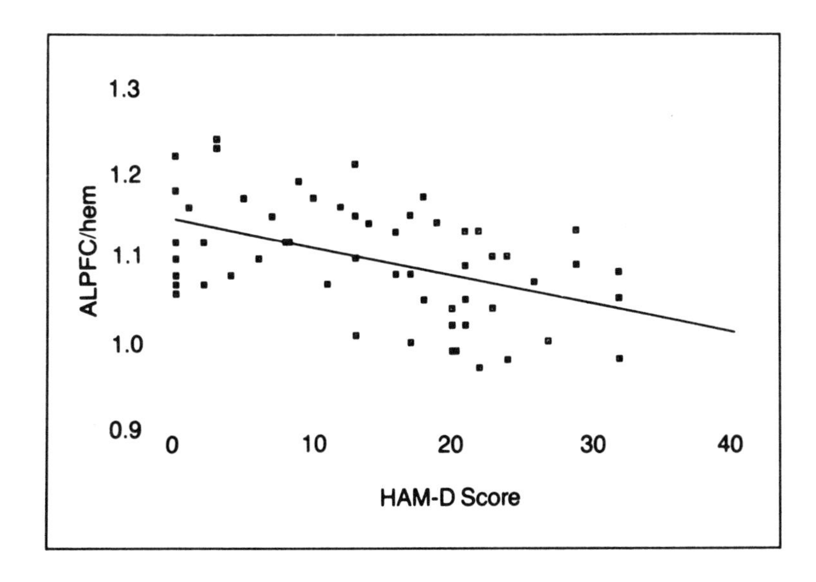

Figure 3-4. Significant correlation between glucose metabolic rates for left middle frontal gyrus (dorsal anterolateral prefrontal cortex), divided by rate for entire hemisphere (ALPFC/hem), and 17-item Hamilton Depression Rating Scale (HAM-D) scores of all subjects at time of study ($r = -.49$; $P = .0002$). Reprinted with permission from Baxter LR, Schwartz JM, Phelps ME, et al: Reduction of prefrontal cortex glucose metabolism common to three types of depression. Arch Gen Psychiatry 46:243–250, 1989. Copyright 1989 American Medical Association.

Post et al. (1987) concluded that temporal lobe activation or a seizure-like process is not occurring during depression. Compared to controls, the depressed patients had significantly reduced relative maximum glucose utilization in right temporal cortex compared to other brain areas in the same slice. They noted these findings were consistent with those of Baxter et al. (1985). Post et al. felt that alternations in left-right temporal lobe metabolic rates would appear to be an area for further investigation in light of the wealth of data, utilizing a variety of methodologies, indicating a role for hemispheric laterality in affective disorders.

PET STUDIES OF BRAIN AMINO ACID POOLS IN MOOD DISORDERS

The carbon 11 (^{11}C) glucose method can be utilized to demonstrate amino acid pools (see Table 3-2). This method has been used to examine amino acid pools in mood disorders (Kishimoto et al. 1987). More than 80% of the activity in the brain seen in images derived from ^{11}C glucose is associated with amino acids such as glutamic acid, glutamine, aspartic acid, gamma-aminobutyric acid, and alanine. In this project, nine unipolar depressed patients were compared to three manic patients, three patients in remission from depression, and seven normal control subjects.

All subjects were right handed, in good physical health (with normal neurologic examinations and laboratory screening examinations), and drug free. All had normal head CT scans. Diagnoses were based on DSM-III criteria and were agreed on by at least two psychiatrists. The nine unipolar depressed patients had no personal or family history suggestive of hypomanic episodes.

In this study, 20 mCi of ^{11}C glucose was administered orally. Subjects were in a room without significant ambient light or auditory stimulation, and their eyes were closed. Initial scans parallel to the orbital meatal line were done 5 minutes after isotope administration. Additional PET images were taken every 10 minutes up to 65 minutes after isotope administration. The PET scanner was a Headtome-II, with a resolution of 11 mm in plane and 12 mm in the axial direction.

The ^{11}C glucose counts in the brain of manic patients were increased about 25% compared to controls (Figure 3-5). The PET images of unipolar depressed patients indicated decreased amino acid pools compared to controls, with ^{11}C counts in the brains of unipolar depressed patients decreased by about 35% compared to controls. The ^{11}C counts in the brains of patients in remission were equivalent to those in normal controls. Amino acid metabolism was examined in frontal, temporal, parietal, and occipital cortices.

There were no differences in the ^{11}C blood counts for controls or patients. Indeed, the uptake of ^{11}C glucose from the blood to the brain was similar in all populations. Therefore, this did not appear to be an explanation for the differences observed among the groups.

There was a disturbed amino acid pool in the cortex of unipolar and bipolar patients. ^{11}C glucose, when employed in the method of Kishimoto et al. (1987), shows amino acid pools, whereas the ^{18}F-deoxyglucose method shows the utilization of glucose itself. These differences in the behavior of the isotopically labeled compounds would explain the difference between their results and those of Buchsbaum et al. (1986) and of Baxter et al. (1985) where the FDG technique was used.

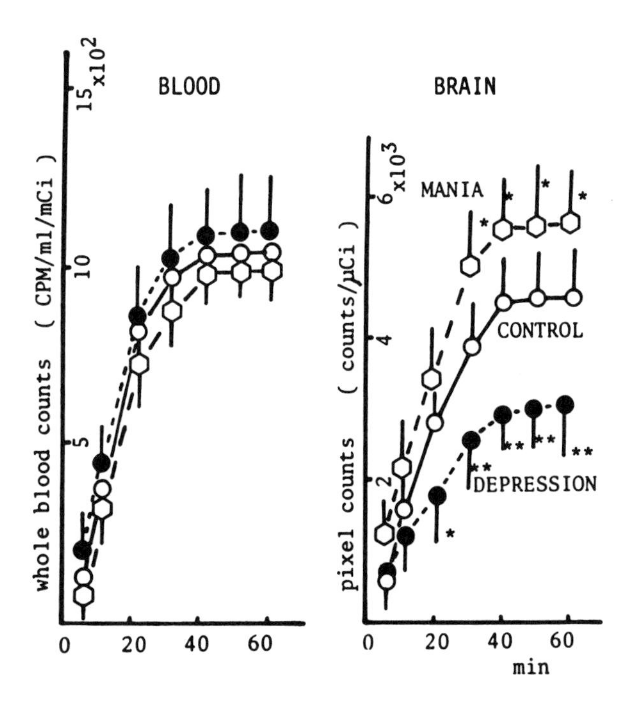

Figure 3-5. ^{11}C counts in blood and brain (frontal) in control, manic, and depressed subjects. Data are presented as means ± SD. Significantly different by *t* test: $^{*}P < .05$; $^{**}P < .01$. Reprinted with permission from Kishimoto H, Takazu O, Ohno S, et al: 11C-Glucose metabolism in manic and depressed patients. Psychiatry Res 22:81–88, 1987. Copyright 1987 Elsevier Scientific Publishers Ireland Ltd.

PET AND BRAIN CIRCULATION

Five patients with major depression received an examination of brain circulation and metabolism (Raichle et al. 1985; see Table 3-2). Four subjects met criteria for major depression according to DSM-III. One subject was a depressed bipolar patient. Subjects were severely depressed, with a mean pretreatment 17-item Hamilton Rating Scale for Depression score of 27 (range, 22–32). The control subjects for the study were normal volunteers.

Subjects were studied using the PETT VI tomograph. ^{15}O-labeled water was used to measure CBF, and ^{15}O-labeled carbon monoxide was used as the tracer to measure cerebral blood volume (CBV). The measurement of local cerebral metabolic rate for oxygen ($CMRO_2$) combines the data obtained from the measurement of CBF and CBV with data obtained from a single inhalation of air containing trace quantities of ^{15}O-labeled molecular oxygen.

CBF and $CMRO_2$ were significantly decreased in patients with depression, compared to normal controls. CBV did not differ significantly from the normal controls.

The authors noted that the data obtained in their study must be considered preliminary and interpreted with caution. The number of patients was small. In addition, all but one of the patients were taking one or more medications prior to being studied.

PET AND SEROTONIN

Spiperone is a potent dopamine D_2 receptor ligand. It is also a serotonin S_2 ligand. Mayberg et al. (1988) imaged cortical serotonin receptor binding using spiperone tagged with ^{11}C (see Table 3-2). Higher S_2 serotonin receptor binding was reported in the right parietal and temporal cortex of 9 patients with right hemisphere strokes when compared to 8 patients with left hemisphere strokes or to 17 normal control subjects (Mayberg et al. 1988). The ratio of binding in the cortex ipsilateral to the stroke versus the contralateral cortex showed a significant negative correlation, with severity for depression in the left temporal cortex. These patients were suffering from an organic mood disorder: poststroke depression. These findings suggest that the biochemical response of the brain may be different depending on which hemisphere is injured and that some depressions may be a consequence of the failure to up-regulate serotonin receptors after stroke.

DISCUSSION

To date, PET findings in mood disorders come from relatively few studies that have used widely different methods, making cross-study interpretations difficult. In fact, only in the case of FDG has there been more than one group reporting anything even approaching similar experiments. Although the investigations of Buchsbaum et al. (1986) and Baxter et al. (1985) could be interpreted as showing similar findings in lateral prefrontal cortex, and both groups reported basal ganglia glucose metabolic dysfunction in various types of depression, a clear picture does not emerge. It should be pointed out that all experiments reviewed here were designed to examine different questions. Nevertheless, it is lamentable that there have been no true replication attempts of any PET mood disorders experiments published as of this writing. This is in contrast to studies of schizophrenia (Buchsbaum et al. 1982; Cohen et al. 1987; Farkas et al. 1984; Jernigan et al. 1985; Kling et al. 1986; Volkow et al. 1986; Wolkin et al. 1988) and even studies of OCD (Baxter et al. 1987, 1988; Nordahl et al. 1989; Swedo et al. 1989), where replication studies within groups and near-replication studies between groups have been reported, allowing a better estimation of "the truth" than is possible for PET mood disorder studies at this time.

There are problems associated with PET in particular, and with studies of psychopathology in general, that are obstacles in all of these studies of mood disorders. These problems can be divided into four areas: 1) patient selection and classification, 2) assessment of patient internal and external conditions at time of study, 3) PET instrumentation and biochemical calculations, and 4) statistical problems.

Patient selection and classification. Mood symptoms of many types are common in the general population, and selecting subjects with homogeneous syndromes on one salient variable (primary diagnosis), while excluding an uncontrolled representation of comorbid pathology (secondary diagnosis) in the same sample, is difficult. All study samples examined have been "convenience samples"—drawn from those presenting at a particular institution—rather than true random samples of the general disease population. Thus results cannot be generalized safely, and significant site-to-site sample differences are likely.

Further, different depressive diseases may manifest similar symptoms. In this regard, an individual may go for many years classified as unipolar, only to have a late-life manic episode and thus switch polarity. Selection of "normal" controls is also a problem with the high prevalence of psychiatric disorders in the general population and the relative ease with which many symptoms can be concealed. Those presenting for studies may be sicker than the general population (Amori and Lenox 1989). Structured diagnostic interviews and diagnosis criteria help but do not eliminate the problem, especially when it comes to the question of meaningful subtypes.

Finally, individuals with mood disorders often show spontaneous state changes over time—more so than is typical of other illnesses, such as schizophrenia. Season and even time of day (Bartlett et al. 1988) may also be important variables, not to mention history of drug exposure. Subtle differences in diagnostic groups samples, as well as mood and other state variations, even within the same individual, may well give differing results.

Assessment of patient internal and external conditions at time of study. It is well demonstrated that alterations in sensory input from the environment to the subject can produce large focal changes in glucose metabolism (Phelps et al. 1986). The studies reported here used a wide range of stimulation states, such as eyes or ears open or closed, nonspecific resting state, and electrical shocks to the arm. At first glance the solution might seem to employ specific behavioral tasks, with a quantifiable behavioral output with which to measure the subject's involvement with the process. However, Mazziotta et al. (1982a, 1982b) demonstrated that, even in the same behavioral task (music memory) and with the same behavioral outcome (scores on memory for a musical sequence), normal individuals using different internal, covert strategies to solve a problem (silent humming versus musical notation) activate different brain areas (right versus left temporal cortex). Thus a psychiatric patient doing a task, such as the Wisconsin Card Sorting Test (Heaton 1985), which usually activates the lateral prefrontal cortex in normals (Weinberger et al. 1986), may fail to activate this same area not because of any problem in the brain structure itself, but because the psychiatric subject chooses to think about the problem in an unusual way. The difference obtained on testing between patient and control subjects may have nothing to do with the basic neural dysfunction in the disease, but rather may reflect a difference in psychology determined by another, unidentified brain region. Even the question of what would be a relevant task for both mood-disordered patients and controls—one that elicits the critical pathology, involves the relevant circuits, and gives an accurate and meaningful behavioral measure—is not clear.

Regardless of the range of states represented in a subject group, simply documenting the subject's mood state at the time of scanning can itself be problematic. Most studies report mood scores for the episode on an instrument like the Hamilton Rating Scale for Depression, but exact mood at time of scanning is rarely documented. Likewise, degree of anxiety is rarely reported. One approach might be to have subjects completing various mood inventories at the time of scanning, but this maneuver in and of itself might perturb cerebral processes and in different ways in different experimental and control groups by processes that have to do with psychological mind set, but not primary psychopathology.

PET instrumentation and biochemical calculations. The intrinsic resolution and time-response capacities of various tomographs, the merits of measured versus calculated attenuation corrections and arterial versus "arterialized" venous blood, the advantages and disadvantages of the particular tracers used, and so on are beyond the scope of this brief review. Interested readers are referred to Phelps et al. (1986). Suffice it to say that all of these factors vary across the studies reviewed.

More fundamental, the meaning of several measures of spiperone binding relative to certain brain reference structures has been questioned even for the D_2 receptor, where there is an affinity much higher than that for the serotonin receptor. Since both serotonin and D_2 receptors are found in the temporal cortex, the relevance of spiperone binding to actual densities of serotonin receptors is open to question. Even PET-FDG, the best validated and most used of all present PET methods (Bartlett et al. 1988; Brooks et al. 1987; Phelps et al. 1986), has uncertainties. Although there is general agreement on glucose metabolic rate value results for the normal human brain, calculations of absolute metabolic rates vary by approximately 10%, even in the same individual in the nonspecific stimulation state done at different times on consecutive days with the same machine and technique (Bartlett et al. 1988). When regional values are "normalized" to whole-brain rates, however, the variation is on the order of only 1% (Bartlett et al. 1988). Whether the time-to-time intrasubject variations observed for absolute metabolic rates are a true reflection of nature or are due to inaccuracies of the method is not clear. However, it must be acknowledged that many of the most problematic variables in the calculation of absolute glucose metabolic rates divide out when normalization is carried out. However, even though the brain is an interactive organ, the exact meaning of normalized metabolic rates is itself not clear (Clark et al. 1989). This would be a problem even if all groups used the same normalization procedure, which they do not.

Statistical problems. Comparing experiments, if the same results are found in different studies, the chance of false-positive (Type I) error may be low, but obviously the risk of false-negative (Type II) error is great in the small sample studies that characterize a complicated, expensive technique such as PET. Within individual experiments, multiple comparisons of many brain regions that are not totally independent are often undertaken, making the probability of Type I error hard to calculate, while multivariate methods used to control for multiple differences among subjects of necessity increases Type II error. Most PET studies of psychiatric illnesses to date are a statistician's nightmare—many approaches to the data analyses can be argued, all giving different results.

PET studies of mood disorders are still in their infancy. Given the high prevalence of mood disorders, and their great costs in both human and economic terms, there will surely be much more of this work in the next few years. Studies of neuroreceptor systems would seem particularly promising.

REFERENCES

American Psychiatric Association: Diagnostic and Statistical Manual of Mental Disorders, 3rd Edition. Washington, DC, American Psychiatric Association, 1980

Amori G. Lenox RH: Do volunteer subjects bias clinical trials? J Clin Psychopharmacol 9:321–327, 1989

Bartlett EJ, Brodie JD, Wolf AP, et al: Reproducibility of cerebral glucose metabolic measurements in resting human subjects. J Cereb Blood Flow Metab 8:502–512, 1988

Baxter LR, Phelps ME, Mazziotta JC, et al: Cerebral metabolic rates for glucose in mood disorders. Arch Gen Psychiatry 42:441–447, 1985

Baxter LR, Phelps ME, Mazziotta JC, et al: Local cerebral glucose metabolic rates in obsessive-compulsive disorder: a comparison with rates in unipolar depression and in normal controls. Arch Gen Psychiatry 44:211–218, 1987

Baxter LR, Schwartz JC, Mazziotta JC, et al: Cerebral glucose metabolic rates in non-depressed obsessive-compulsives. Am J Psychiatry 145: 1560–1563, 1988

Baxter LR, Schwartz JM, Phelps ME, et al: Reduction of prefrontal cortex glucose metabolism common to three types of depression. Arch Gen Psychiatry 46:243–250, 1989

Brooks RA, Hatazawa J, Chiro GD, et al: Human cerebral glucose metabolism determined by positron emission tomography: a revisit. J Cereb Blood Flow Metab 7:427–432, 1987

Buchsbaum M, Ingvar D, Kessler R, et al: Cerebral glucography with positron tomography: use in normal subjects and in patients with schizophrenia. Arch Gen Psychiatry 39:251–259, 1982

Buchsbaum MS, DeLisi LE, Holomb HH, et al: Anteroposterior gradients in cerebral glucose use in schizophrenia and affective disorders. Arch Gen Psychiatry 41:1159–1166, 1984

Buchsbaum MS, Wu J, DeLisi LE, et al: Frontal cortex and basal ganglia metabolic rates assessed by positron emission tomography with [18F] 2-deoxyglucose in affective illness. J Affective Disord 10:137–152, 1986

Clark C, Klonoff H, Tyhurst JS, et al: Regional cerebral glucose metabolism in three sets of identical twins with psychotic symptoms. Can J Psychiatry 34:263–270, 1989

Cohen R, Semple W, Gross M, et al: Dysfunction in a prefrontal substrate of sustained attention in schizophrenia. Life Sci 40:2031–2039, 1987

Endicott J, Spitzer RL: A diagnostic interview: the Schedule for Affective Disorders and Schizophrenia. Arch Gen Psychiatry 35:837–844, 1978

Farkas T, Wolf A, Jaeger J, et al: Regional brain glucose metabolism in chronic schizophrenia. Arch Gen Psychiatry 41:293–300, 1984

Gustafson L, Risberg J, Silfverskiold P: Regional cerebral blood flow in organic dementia and affective disorders. Advances in Biological Psychiatry 6:109–116, 1981

Hamilton M: Development of a rating scale for primary depressive illness. Br J Soc Psychol 6:278–296, 1967

Heaton R: Wisconsin Card Sorting Test. Odessa, TX, Psychological Assessment Resources, 1985

Huang SC, Phelps ME, Hoffman EJ, et al: Non-invasive determination of local cerebral metabolic rate of glucose in man. Am J Physiol 238:E69–E82, 1980

Jernigan T, Sargent T, Pfefferbaum A, et al: Fluorodeoxyglucose PET in schizophrenia. Psychiatry Res 16:317–329, 1985

Kishimoto H, Takazu O, Ohno S, et al: 11C-Glucose metabolism in manic and depressed patients. Psychiatry Res 22:81–88, 1987

Kling A, Metter J, Riege W, et al: Comparison of PET measurement of local brain glucose metabolism and CAT measurement of brain atrophy in chronic schizophrenia and depression. Am J Psychiatry 143:175–180, 1986

Mathew RJ, Mayer JS, Frances DJ, et al: Cerebral blood flow in depression. Am J Psychiatry 137:1449–1450, 1980

Matsui T, Hirano A: An Atlas of the Human Brain for Computerized Tomography. Tokyo, Igaku-Shoin, 1978

Mayberg HS, Robinson RG, Wong DF, et al: PET imaging of cortical S2 serotonin receptors after stroke: lateralized changes in relationship to depression. Am J Psychiatry 145:937–943, 1988

Mazziotta JC, Phelps ME, Carson RE, et al: Tomographic mapping of human cerebral metabolism: auditory stimulation. Neurology 32:921–937, 1982a

Mazziotta JC, Phelps ME, Carson RE, et al: Tomographic mapping of human cerebral metabolism: sensory deprivation. Ann Neurol 12:435–444, 1982b

Nordahl TE, Benkelfat C, Semple WE, et al: Cerebral glucose metabolic rates in obsessive-compulsive disorder. Neuropsychopharmacology 2:23–28, 1989

Phelps ME, Huang SC, Hoffman EJ, et al: Tomographic measurement of local cerebral glucose metabolic rate in humans with (F18) 2-fluoro-2-deoxyglucose: validation of method. Ann Neurol 6:371–388, 1979

Phelps ME, Mazziotta JC, Gerner R, et al: Human cerebral glucose metabolism in affective disorders: drug-free states and pharmacologic effects. J Cereb Blood Flow Metab 3(Suppl):S7–S8, 1983

Phelps ME, Mazziotta JC, Baxter L, et al: Study design in the investigation of mood disorders with PET, in Brain Imaging and Brain Function. Edited by Sokoloff L. New York, Raven, 1985, pp 227–243

Phelps ME, Mazziotta JC, Schelbert HR: Positron Emission Tomography and Autoradiography: Principles and Application for the Brain. New York, Raven, 1986

Post RM, DeLisi LE, Holcomb HH, et al: Glucose utilization in the temporal cortex of affectively ill patients: positron emission tomography. Biol Psychiatry 22:545–553, 1987

Raichle ME, Taylor JR, Herscovtch P, et al: Brain circulation and metabolism and depression, in The Metabolism of the Human Brain Studied with Positron Emission Tomography. Edited by Greitz T, et al. New York, Raven, 1985, pp 453–456

Rush AJ, Schlessor MA, Stokley E, et al: Cerebral blood flow in depression and mania, in Brain Imaging in Psychiatry and Neurology: Positron Emission Tomography and Other Techniques. Edited by Buchsbaum MS, Eusdin E, Bunney Jr WE, et al. Pacific Grove, CA, Boxwood Press, 1982

Sokoloff L: Relation between physiological function and energy metabolism in the central nervous system. J Neurochem 29:13–26, 1977

Swedo SE, Schapiro MB, Grady CL, et al: Cerebral glucose metabolism in childhood-onset obsessive-compulsive disorder. Arch Gen Psychiatry 46:518–523, 1989

Volkow N, Brodie J, Wolf A, et al: Brain organization of schizophrenics. J Cereb Blood Flow Metab 6:441–446, 1986

Weinberger DR, Beman KF, Zee RF: Physiologic dysfunction of dorsolateral prefrontal cortex in schizophrenia, I: regional blood flow evidence. Arch Gen Psychiatry 43:114–124, 1986

Wolkin A, Angrist B, Wolf A, et al: Low frontal glucose utilization in chronic schizophrenia: a replication study. Am J Psychiatry 145:251–253, 1988

Chapter 4

Structural Brain Abnormalities in the Depressed Elderly

C. Edward Coffey, M.D.

Magnetic resonance imaging (MRI) uses radio-frequency radiation in the presence of a magnetic field to create cross-sectional images of the body. In addition to providing highly accurate anatomic detail, MRI is also a very sensitive technique for detecting abnormal tissue or changes in tissue composition. Over the past several years we have conducted a series of clinical and research studies using high-field-strength MRI to investigate abnormalities of brain tissue and structure in elderly patients with depression. Our studies have focused primarily on severely depressed patients referred for electroconvulsive therapy (ECT) in an effort to examine the impact of preexisting structural brain abnormalities on the therapeutic and adverse effects of ECT. In this chapter, I will provide a summary of our findings and review their potential clinical and pathophysiologic implications.

EARLY RETROSPECTIVE DATA

In an early series of case reports and retrospective clinical studies that utilized computed tomography (CT) and brain MRI, we found that structural brain abnormalities were surprisingly common in 67 elderly (≥60 years) depressed patients referred for ECT (Coffey et al. 1987, 1988a, 1988b; Figiel et al. 1989). The most common abnormalities included cortical atrophy (69%), lateral ventricular enlargement (67%), and subcortical hyperintensity (i.e., foci of T2 hyperintensity in the subcortical white matter and deep gray nuclei) (67%). Most patients had various combinations of these findings. In patients who

Supported by grants from the National Institute of Mental Health (MH41803, MH30723, and MH40159), the National Institutes of Health (M01-RR-30), and the North Carolina United Way. The author gratefully acknowledges a number of colleagues who assisted with various aspects of this work: W.T. Djang, G.S. Figiel, P. Holt, W.B. Saunders, J. Shavender, S. Soady, M. Webb, R.D. Weiner, and W.E. Wilkinson.

received both MRI and CT, the MRI study frequently revealed changes not visible on the CT scan.

Of clinical interest, 58% of the patients with structural brain abnormalities did not develop their first episode of depression until after the age of 60 ("late-age-onset depression"). Furthermore, despite extensive brain changes in some patients, dementia was uncommon. The majority of patients showed a good clinical response to their course of ECT, and major adverse cognitive effects (i.e., prolonged disorientation, complaints of persistent memory disturbances) were uncommon.

Although intriguing, the clinical significance of these findings was limited by the retrospective study design and by the absence of a normal control group. Subsequently, prospective clinical studies were undertaken to compare the prevalence and severity of structural brain abnormalities in a new group of 51 elderly depressed subjects referred for ECT to a normal control group of 22 elderly subjects with no history of neurologic or psychiatric illness. Additional details of these subject populations have been previously reported (Coffey and Figiel, in press; Coffey et al. 1989, 1990).

CONTROLLED PROSPECTIVE INVESTIGATIONS

Brain MRI Procedure

All brain MRI studies were performed on a General Electric 1.5 Tesla Signa system. Spin-echo pulse sequences were used to generate both T1 weighted (repetition time [TR] = 500 msec, echo time [TE] = 20 msec), intermediate (TR = 2,500 msec, TE = 40 msec), and T2 weighted (TR = 2,500 msec, TE = 80 msec) images in the axial, coronal, and sagittal planes. Images were 5 mm thick, with a 2.5-mm interscan gap. Typical technical parameters included a 128 × 256 matrix, 20-cm field of view, and two excitations.

The brain MRI scans were analyzed independently by a board-certified neuroradiologist and a neurologist/psychiatrist, both of whom were blind to subject group (depressed or control) and to the clinical interpretation of each study. Using formal rating instruments suited to MRI, each patient's MRI study was assessed for the presence and extent of the following findings.

Cortical atrophy. A cortical atrophy score was determined from a 5-point rating scale: 0 = no atrophy, 1 = slight atrophy, 2 = mild atrophy, 3 = moderate atrophy, and 4 = severe atrophy (Largen et al. 1984). Predefined visual standards for each grade were established for comparison (Figure 4-1). The cortical atrophy score for each patient was defined as the average score of the two raters (fractions were rounded to the nearest integer). Any left-right asymmetries were also recorded.

Lateral ventricular enlargement. A lateral ventricular enlargement score was determined from a 5-point rating scale: 0 = no enlargement, 1 = slight enlargement, 2 = mild enlargement, 3 = moderate enlargement, and 4 = severe enlargement (Drayer et al. 1985). Ventricular enlargement was rated only if it was considered to be more extensive than would be expected for the patient's age (for an example, see Figure 4-1). The lateral ventricular enlargement score for each patient was defined as the average score of the two raters, and fractions were rounded to the nearest integer. Any left-right asymmetries were also recorded.

Subcortical hyperintensity (including periventricular hyperintensity and deep white matter hyperintensity). Both periventricular hyperintensity and deep white matter hyperintensity were rated separately for each hemisphere from the intermediate and T2 weighted axial images, using a modification of the 4-point scale described by Fazekas et al. (1987). Periventricular hyperintensity was graded as 0 = absent, 1 = "caps" or pencil-thin lining, 2 = smooth "halo," and 3 = irregular periventricular hyperintensity extending into the deep white matter. Separate deep white matter hyperintensity changes were rated as 0 = absent, 1 = punctate foci, 2 = beginning confluence of foci, and 3 = large confluent areas. Predefined visual standards for each grade were established for comparison (Figures 4-2 and 4-3). Changes in the subcortical gray matter nuclei (basal ganglia, thalamus) were rated as punctate, multipunctate, or diffuse, and any left-right asymmetries were noted (Figure 4-4).

In the event of disagreement between raters with respect to abnormalities of the subcortical white matter or gray matter nuclei, the scans were reanalyzed and a consensus rating was established by the two raters.

Prevalence and Severity of Structural Brain Abnormalities

Cortical atrophy. Cortical atrophy (mild or greater) was found in 96% (49 of 51) of the elderly depressed subjects referred for ECT who received brain MRI at Duke University Medical Center in 1987 (Table 4-1). The cortical atrophy appeared to be especially severe in the 16 patients with a known history of neurologic illness (e.g., dementia, cerebrovascular disease, Parkinson's disease). Still, comparing only those depressed subjects *without* any evidence of neurologic illness, at least moderately severe ($\geq$ grade 3) cortical atrophy was significantly more common ($\chi^2 = 5.79$, 1 df, $P = .02$) in the depressed group (17 of 35, 49%) than in the normal controls (3 of 22, 14%).

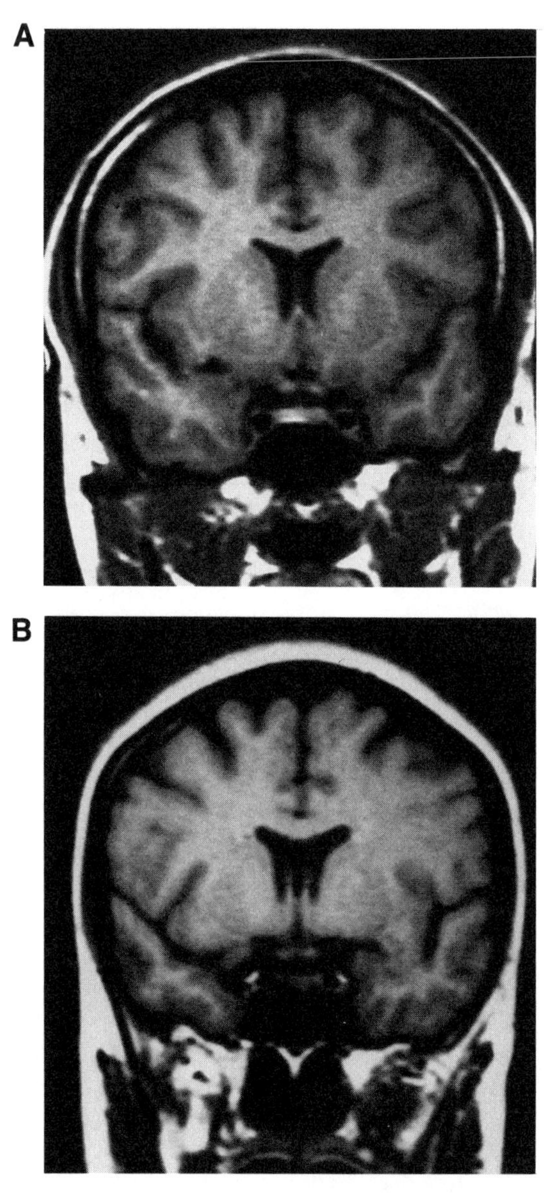

Figure 4-1. Visual standards for cortical atrophy score (CAS) ratings on T1 weighted coronal magnetic resonance imaging: *A:* CAS = 0,1 (none, borderline); *B:* CAS = 2 (mild cortical atrophy).

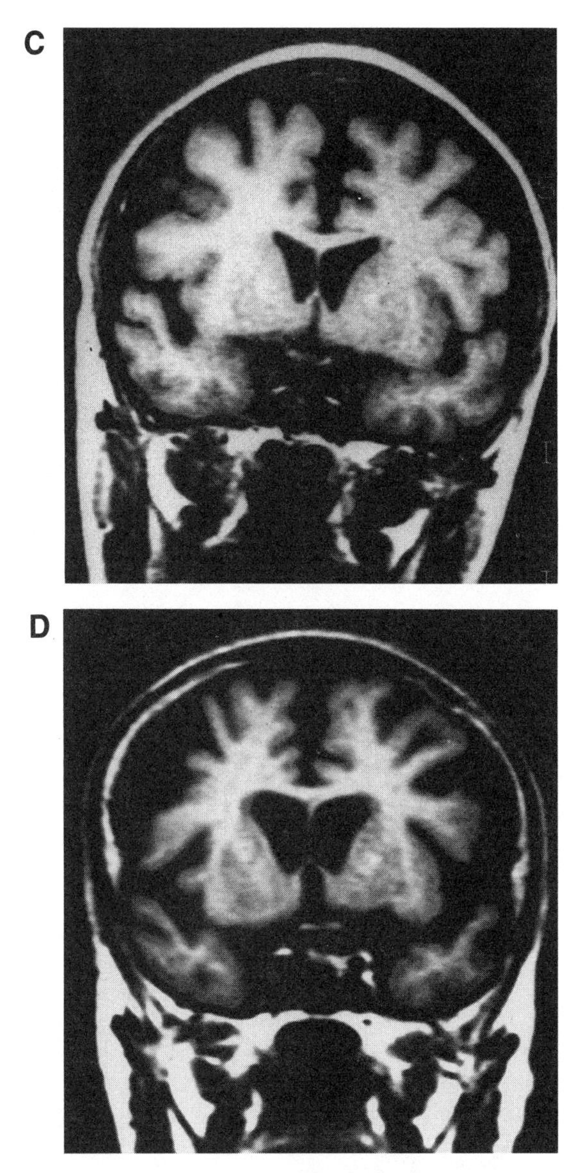

Figure 4-1 (*continued*). *C:* CAS = 3 (moderate cortical atrophy, with widening of the interhemispheric fissure); *D:* CAS = 4 (severe cortical atrophy, with widening of almost all sulci; this subject also exhibits enlargement of the lateral ventricles).

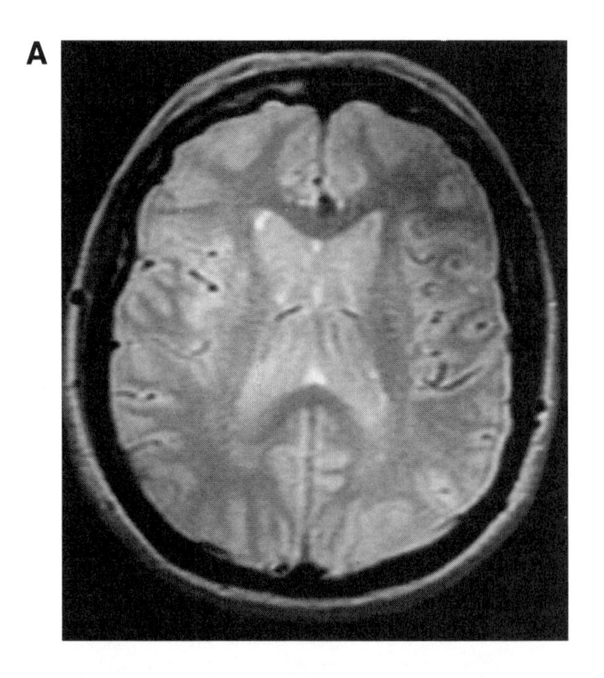
A

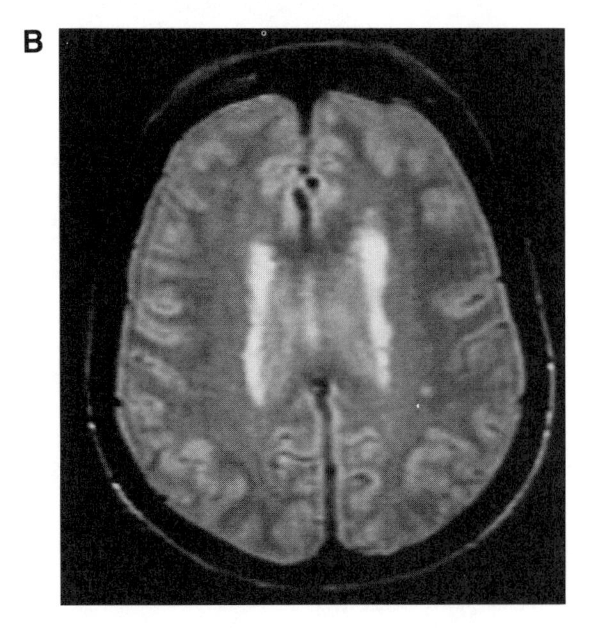
B

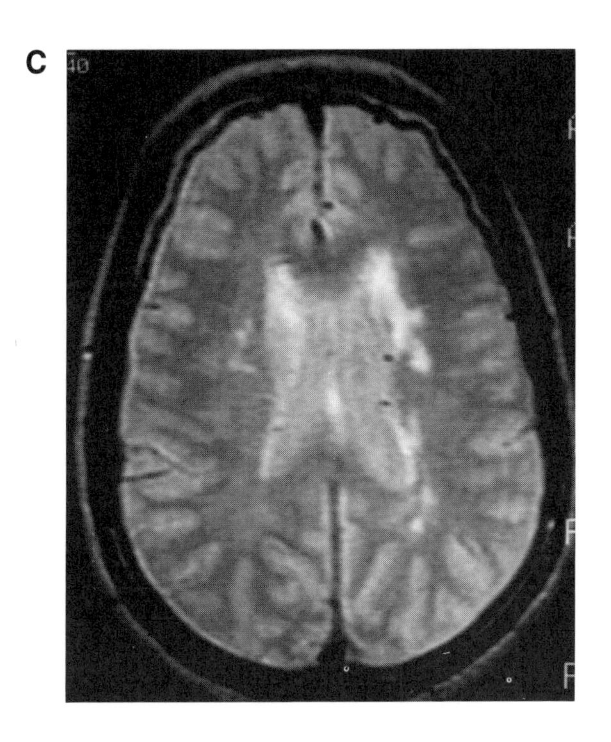

Figure 4-2. Visual standards for periventricular hyperintensity (PVH) on magnetic resonance imaging (repetition time [TR] = 2,500 msec, echo time [TE] = 80 msec): *A:* Grade 1 PVH, "caps" at anterior tips of frontal horns; *B:* Grade 2 PVH, "halo" along border of lateral ventricles; *C:* Grade 3 PVH, irregular extension of hyperintensity into the deep white matter.

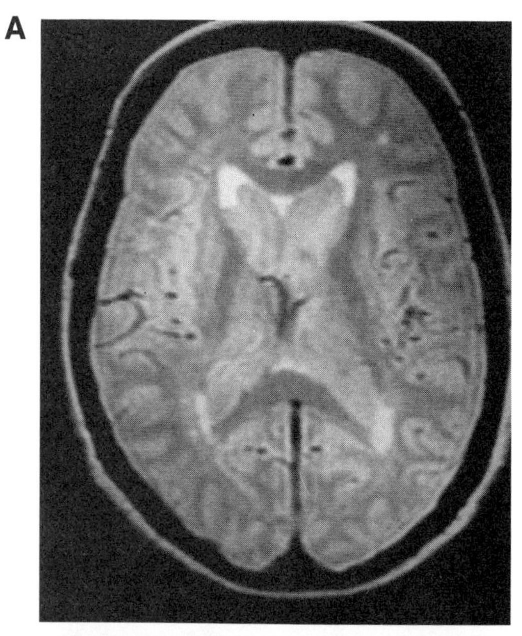
A

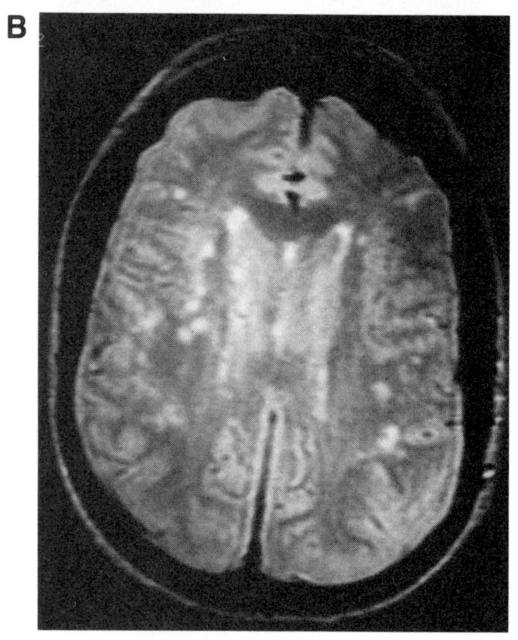
B

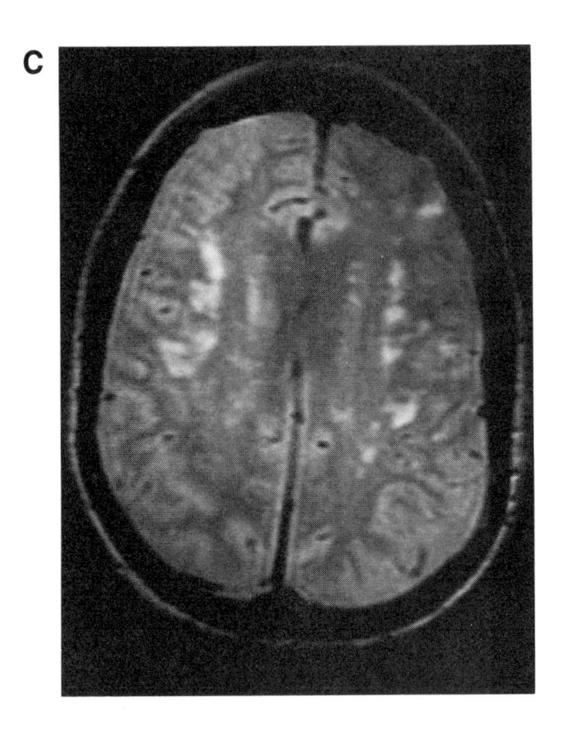

Figure 4-3. Visual standards for deep white matter hyperintensity (DWMH) on magnetic resonance imaging (repetition time [TR] = 2,500 msec, echo time [TE] = 80 msec): *A:* Grade 1 DWMH, punctate focus; *B:* Grade 2 DWMH, small confluence of foci; *C:* Grade 3 DWMH, large confluent areas of DWMH.

These findings are consistent with a small number of previous reports using CT (Dolan et al. 1986; Kolbeinsson et al. 1986) and demonstrate that cortical atrophy is common in the depressed elderly.

Lateral ventricular enlargement. Lateral ventricular enlargement (mild or greater) was seen in 69% (35 of 51) of our depressed subjects, and it appeared to be most severe in those patients with a history of neurologic illness. Ventriculomegaly was also seen in 63% of depressed subjects without neurologic disease, although its prevalence did not differ significantly (χ^2 = 1.81, 1 df, P = .18) from that of the normal controls (41%).

Subcortical hyperintensity. With respect to subcortical hyperintensity, predominantly mild changes were observed in all normal control subjects (Table 4-1) (Coffey et al. 1990). Periventricular caps (grade 1) were seen in 17 of the 22 (77%) normal controls, and the remaining 5 (23%) exhibited a more or less smooth halo (grade 2) of peri-

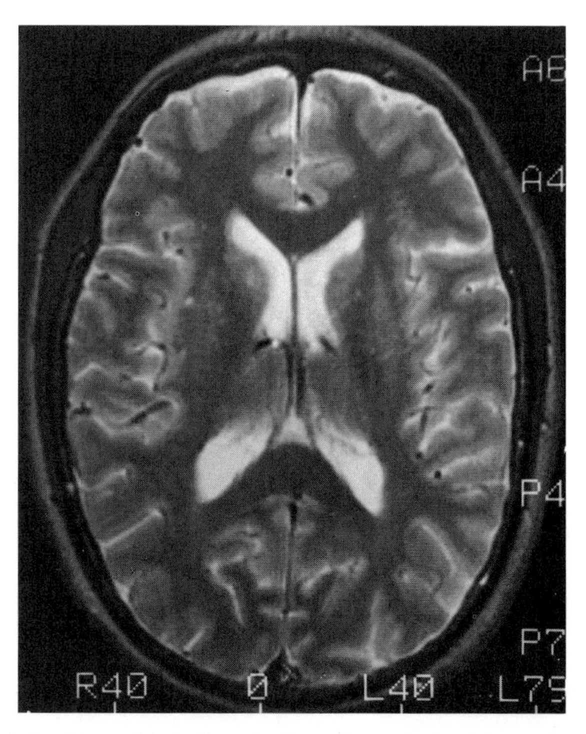

Figure 4-4. Example of subcortical hyperintensity in right caudate nucleus on magnetic resonance imaging (repetition time [TR] = 2,500 msec, echo time [TE] = 80 msec).

ventricular hyperintensity. Separate foci of T2 hyperintensity in the deep white matter were also seen in 17 of the 22 (77%) normal subjects. These changes appeared either as punctate foci (grade 1) (64%) or as areas of small confluence (grade 2) (13%). No normal subject exhibited severe (grade 3) periventricular or deep white matter hyperintensity. Foci of T2 hyperintensity in the subcortical gray nuclei were observed in only 1 (5%) of the normal controls. These findings are in close agreement with previous studies that have examined the prevalence and severity of subcortical hyperintensity in a small number of normal subjects (Coffey and Figiel, in press; Fazekas et al. 1987; George et al. 1986).

Subcortical hyperintensity was also present in all of the depressed subjects, but the changes were more severe than in the control group (Coffey and Figiel, in press; Coffey et al. 1990) (Table 4-1). Comparing only those 35 depressed subjects *without* any history of neurologic illness, moderate plus severe periventricular hyperintensity was significantly more common ($\chi^2 = 4.9$, 1 df, $P = .03$) in the depressed group (57%) than in the controls (23%). Moderate plus severe deep white matter hyperintensity was also significantly more common ($\chi^2 = 5.18$, 1 df, $P = .02$) in the depressed group (46%) than in the controls (13%). Similarly, lesions of the thalamus/basal ganglia were significantly more common (Fisher's exact test, $P = .003$) in the depressed patients (40%) than in the normal control population (5%).

These data demonstrate that subcortical hyperintensity is more common and more severe in elderly depressed patients (at least those referred for ECT) than in a normal control population with similar age and prevalence of vascular disease. Our findings also demonstrate the importance of using formal rating scales to assess the severity and extent of subcortical hyperintensity. For example, no differences between our elderly depressed and control subjects would have been revealed if the comparisons had been based solely on the neuroradiologist's clinical report of the presence or absence of foci of subcortical hyperintensity.

For both the control and depressed groups, the severity of subcortical hyperintensity appeared to be related to the presence of risk factors for vascular disease. Among the control subjects, for example, moderate periventricular hyperintensity appeared to be more common in subjects with vascular disease (4 of 14, 29%) than in those without vascular disease (1 of 8, 13%), and every subject with either moderate deep white matter hyperintensity ($n = 3$) or lesions of the deep gray nuclei ($n = 1$) had vascular disease. Similarly, depressed subjects with a history of neurologic illness had the highest prevalence rates of moderate plus severe subcortical hyperintensity (Table 4-1),

Table 4-1. Prevalence of clinical and brain magnetic resonance imaging findings in normal elderly control subjects and elderly inpatients with major depression referred for electroconvulsive therapy

Characteristic	Normal controls (n = 22)		Depressed inpatients: No neurologic history (n = 35)		Depressed inpatients: Neurologic history (n = 16)		Depressed inpatients: Total (n = 51)	
	n	%	n	%	n	%	n	%
Age (mean ± SD years)	70.7 ± 5.5		71.7 ± 8.1		71.7 ± 6.8		71.7 ± 7.7	
Vascular risk factors								
Male sex	7	32	7	20	8	50	15	29
Hypertension	3	14	8	23	6	38	14	27
Diabetes mellitus	1	5	0		1	6	1	2
Coronary artery disease	7	32	5	14	3	19	8	16
Stroke	0		0		7	44	7	14
Cortical atrophy								
1 (Borderline)	4	18	2	6	0		2	4
2 (Mild)	15	68	16	46	3	19	19	37
3 (Moderate)	3	14	12	34	9	56	21	41
4 (Severe)	0		5	14	3	19	8	16
Lateral ventricular enlargement								
2 (Mild)	5	23	15	43	5	31	20	39
3 (Moderate)	4	18	7	20	6	38	13	25
4 (Severe)	0		0		2	13	2	4

Periventricular hyperintensity								
Grade 1	17	77	15	43	4	25	19	37
Grade 2	5	23	15	43	4	25	19	37
Grade 3	0		5	14	8	50	13	26
Deep white matter hyperintensity								
None	5	23	6	17	1	6	7	14
Grade 1	14	64	13	37	3	19	16	31
Grade 2	3	14	10	29	6	38	16	31
Grade 3	0		6	17	6	38	12	24
Lesions of the thalamus/basal ganglia	1	5	14	40	12	75	26	51

and even among subjects with no neurologic history, those with vascular risk factors ($n = 13$) tended to have higher rates of moderate plus severe deep white matter hyperintensity (54% versus 41%) and lesions of the deep gray nuclei (54% versus 32%) than those without vascular disease ($n = 22$), respectively. These findings highlight the critical importance of appropriate control groups. Since the severity of subcortical hyperintensity is related in part to vascular disease (Coffey and Figiel, in press), it is imperative that this variable be considered whenever comparisons among subjects are made. The potential impact of other factors (e.g., smoking, hypercholesterolemia) may also need to be considered (Coffey et al. 1990).

Clinical Correlates of Structural Brain Abnormalities in the Depressed Elderly

There was no association between a history of ECT and the severity of any of the brain MRI abnormalities (Coffey et al. 1989). For example, a history of ECT was found in 11 of 28 (39%) patients with at least moderately severe cortical atrophy (cortical atrophy score ≥3) versus 15 of 22 (68%) patients with less severe atrophy. Similar negative results with CT and MRI have been reported by most others (for a review, see Coffey et al. 1988a), indicating that a causal relationship between ECT and structural brain abnormalities would appear unlikely. Furthermore, the high prevalence of structural brain abnormalities observed in our population of ECT referrals highlights the serious limitations that are inherent in retrospective studies that report associations between prior ECT and current brain imaging abnormalities (Coffey et al. 1988a)—clearly such abnormalities may have been present before ECT.

Although the initial onset of depression in late life appears in general to be uncommon (Dorzab et al. 1971), the majority (81%) of our 51 patients experienced their first episode of affective disorder after the age of 60. Indeed, such late-age-onset depression was seen in 93% of subjects with at least moderately severe cortical atrophy (cortical atrophy score ≥3) and in 100% of subjects with severe (grade 3) periventricular and/or deep white matter hyperintensity ($n = 13$). Although partially confounded by ceiling effects, these data suggest that structural brain abnormalities may be associated with late-age-onset depressive illness.

A preliminary review of symptom data in our 51 depressed patients suggested that major depression with melancholia, as defined by DSM-III criteria (American Psychiatric Association 1980), may be relatively less common in patients with moderate or severe cortical atrophy (59% versus 91% in subjects with lesser atrophy). Shima et al.

(1984) reported similar findings. In addition, psychotic symptoms appeared to be relatively uncommon in patients with lesions in the basal ganglia (15% versus 44% with such lesions). These observations are consistent with recent data suggesting a relationship in depressed patients between psychotic symptoms, structural brain changes, and dopaminergic function in the basal ganglia (Pearlson et al. 1988; Rothschild et al. 1988; Schatzberg et al. 1988). Finally, dementia (DSM-III) that preceded the onset of the index depressive episode was present in 10 of the 51 (20%) patients, and it appeared to be more common in those with subcortical hyperintensity of the deep gray nuclei (38%) than in patients without such lesions (0%). Still, it is of interest that despite extensive cortical and subcortical brain abnormalities in many patients, dementia was uncommon.

An abnormal (nonsuppressed) dexamethasone suppression test (DST) was noted in 18 of the 24 (75%) subjects who received the test prior to ECT. There was no association between DST nonsuppression and the prevalence or severity of any of the structural brain abnormalities. Polysomnographic studies were obtained in 12 of our subjects; rapid eye movement (REM) latency was found to be significantly shorter ($P = .03$) in the 4 subjects with lesions (foci of T2 hyperintensity) in the pons (20.6 min ± 27) than in the 8 subjects without pontine lesions (53.6 min ± 19). Sleep-onset REM was seen in 3 of the 4 (75%) subjects with pontine lesions; none of the remaining 8 subjects with normal pons exhibited sleep-onset REM. These findings are of interest given the hypothesized role of pontine mechanisms in the regulation of REM sleep (Siegel 1989).

The majority (82%) of our 51 patients met criteria for a full therapeutic response to the course of ECT (global clinical rating [Guy 1976] of mildly ill or less 2–3 days after ECT), irrespective of the severity of the structural brain abnormalities (Coffey et al. 1989). For example, the percentage of responders was similar in patients with (23 of 29, 79%) and without (19 of 22, 86%) at least moderately severe subcortical hyperintensity. These findings are consistent with previous reports (Price and McAllister 1989) and suggest that patients with organic brain disease may show a good clinical response to ECT.

The extent to which patients with structural brain abnormalities may be at increased risk for developing cognitive side effects from ECT was difficult to assess in our clinical study, possibly because the test measures were relatively insensitive (Coffey et al. 1989). Still, certain trends were present. With respect to reorientation after the sixth ECT treatment, for example, the percentage of patients with delayed (> 60 min) reorientation was suggestively greater in those with (21%) versus those without (7%) at least moderately severe cortical atrophy. An additional potential relationship between cognitive changes and structural brain abnormalities was demonstrated in regard to the presence of interictal delirium, which developed in five of our patients. Interestingly, lesions of the basal ganglia appeared to be more common in these patients than in those who did not develop delirium (80% versus 48%), a finding consistent with recent data in stroke patients implicating the basal ganglia in poststroke agitated delirium (Caplan et al. 1988; Mori and Yamadori 1987). Still, because our patients with basal ganglia lesions also tended to have more severe cortical and subcortical abnormalities, it is possible that this increased prevalence of delirium may have been a reflection of the overall severity of brain changes in these subjects (Figiel et al. 1990).

DISCUSSION

Only a small number of previous imaging studies have examined cerebral anatomy in the depressed elderly, and results have been contradictory. Prominence of the cortical sulci (Dolan et al. 1986; Kolbeinsson et al. 1986) and increased lateral ventricular brain ratios have been described on CT (Dolan et al. 1985; Jacoby et al. 1983; Yates et al. 1987), although this latter finding has not been confirmed by others (Dolan et al. 1985; Kolbeinsson et al. 1986; Shima et al. 1984). Cerebellar atrophy (Yates et al. 1987) and reductions in brain tissue density (Jacoby et al. 1983) have also been reported in some elderly depressed patients relative to controls. Using high-field-strength MRI, we have found that elderly depressed inpatients referred for ECT exhibit a variety of structural brain abnormalities, including cortical atrophy, subcortical hyperintensity, and lateral ventricular enlargement.

More recently we have begun to extend these studies to include quantitative determinations of the volume of a structure of interest made from contiguous T1 weighted coronal sections of the MRI scans. Similar methods have been used to reveal brain anatomic differences between normal subjects and patients with schizophrenia (Kelsoe et al. 1988; Suddath et al. 1989) or dementia (Seab et al. 1988). The greater sensitivity of this volumetric measure should enhance our ability to detect structural brain abnormalities in our elderly depressed patients. Indeed, preliminary data from our laboratory suggest that total frontal lobe volume is significantly smaller ($t = 2.75$, 29 df, $P < .01$) in a new sample of 14 elderly depressed subjects with no history of neurologic illness (220 ml ± 31) than in a sample of 17 normal elderly controls (250 ml ± 31). In contrast, total temporal lobe volume did not differ significantly between the elderly depressed (98 ml ± 20) and normal control (104 ml ± 16) groups.

These data support our previous clinical findings of cortical atrophy in the depressed elderly and suggest that the atrophy may be relatively specific for the frontal lobes.

The precise etiology of the structural brain abnormalities observed in our elderly depressed population is not known. The cortical atrophy could be related to a variety of medical factors that frequently accompany severe depressive illness in the elderly (e.g., malnutrition, weight loss, neglect of physical health). Drug and alcohol use, which might increase during the depressive episodes, could be an additional contributing factor. It would also be of interest to determine whether cortical atrophy (and especially atrophy of the frontal lobes) is present in younger patients with depression. Findings to date suggest that cortical atrophy may be uncommon in nonelderly patients with depression (Jeste et al. 1988b; Nasrallah et al. 1989), although patients referred specifically for ECT have not been systematically studied. Such investigations, which are currently underway in our laboratory, would allow a determination of whether the sulcal prominence represents an early nonprogressive "dystrophy" or a progressive atrophic process.

Our findings that subcortical hyperintensity is common in depressed patients (at least the elderly) may also provide a potential pathophysiologic explanation for other alterations in brain structure and function reported in depression, including lateral ventricular enlargement (Jeste 1988b; Nasrallah et al. 1989) and reduced glucose metabolism of the caudate nuclei on positron-emission tomography (Baxter et al. 1985). As we have discussed elsewhere (Coffey and Figiel, in press), subcortical hyperintensity on MRI likely reflects a range of neuropathologic changes resulting primarily from ischemia to the subcortical brain regions. It is possible that with progression of this disease process, the periventricular white and gray matter structures might eventually become atrophic, resulting in ex vacuo expansion of the lateral ventricles and a reduction in the regional metabolic activity of the caudate and other periventricular structures. We are beginning to explore these issues with an examination of the relationships between the severity of subcortical hyperintensity on MRI and the size of the periventricular structures as determined by quantitative volumetric analyses. This technical approach should provide important information about the location of brain lesions responsible for ventriculomegaly in elderly patients with depression. Similar investigations should also be performed in nonelderly depressed subjects as well, since lateral ventricular enlargement appears to be common in this population (Jeste et al. 1988b; Nasrallah et al. 1989) and since recent reports suggest that subcortical hyperintensity may also be present in at least some nonelderly depressed patients (Dupont et al. 1990; Krishnan et al. 1988).

Our findings suggest that some of the clinical and biological parameters of depressive illness in the elderly may be related to the presence of structural brain abnormalities. For example, the severity of both the cortical and subcortical abnormalities observed in our depressed group appeared to be related to the development of late-age-onset (after age 60 years) depressive illness (Coffey et al. 1988b, 1989). Similar findings with respect to lateral ventricular enlargement have been described by others (Jacoby and Levy 1980; Rossi et al. 1987; Shima et al. 1984), although Dolan et al. (1986) reported that cortical atrophy was not associated with age at onset. More recent preliminary data have described subcortical hyperintensity in a small number of patients with late-onset schizophrenia (Jeste et al. 1988a) and late-onset atypical psychosis (Miller et al. 1989). Taken together, these data suggest that subjects with structural brain abnormalities (especially subcortical) may be at risk for developing the onset of psychiatric illnesses in late life.

Although the precise pathophysiologic mechanisms for this potential "risk factor" remain speculative, one could hypothesize that diffuse cortical and/or subcortical lesions might disrupt neurotransmitter pathways (e.g., catecholamines, indoleamines) known to course through these areas. A "neurochemical disconnection syndrome" might then result, with regional alterations in neurotransmitter concentration or function producing various disturbances of affect, thought, or cognition. Additional work in elderly subjects is needed to determine more precisely the prevalence and severity of cortical and subcortical lesions and their association with age at onset of affective illness.

It would also be of interest to determine whether particular structural brain abnormalities might be associated with specific clinical symptoms or biological markers of depressive illness in the elderly. In this regard, a preliminary review of our data has suggested that some symptoms (e.g., melancholia, psychosis) may be relatively less common in patients with extensive brain disease, whereas other symptoms (e.g., dementia) may be relatively more common. Furthermore, a potential relationship between structural brain abnormalities and biological markers for depression was suggested by our observation of an apparent association between lesions of the pons on MRI and shortened REM latencies, including sleep-onset REM. Clearly, these data require replication in a larger group of subjects; if confirmed, however, they may provide insights into the neurobiological mechanisms that mediate at least some of the clinical symptoms and laboratory correlates of depression in patients with organic brain disease.

Our finding that structural brain abnormalities are common in depressed patients referred for ECT raises the possibility that such patients may be predisposed toward the type of affective illnesses for which ECT is recommended (Coffey et al. 1988b). For example, there may exist a subgroup of patients with brain MRI abnormalities (e.g., subcortical hyperintensity, cortical atrophy, or ventricular enlargement) who are likely to develop affective illness. Such patients might be relatively refractory to drug therapy and thus referred for ECT, or they might develop especially severe depressions with symptoms that preferentially suggest the use of ECT (e.g., psychosis, incapacitating melancholia). Support for this hypothesis is provided by studies that report associations between structural brain abnormalities on CT (e.g., cortical atrophy, ventricular enlargement) and more prolonged or severe depressive illnesses with psychotic features (reviewed in Jeste et al. 1988b and Nasrallah et al. 1989). If confirmed, such findings could have important implications for the pathophysiology of depressive illness in patients with organic brain disease, and they offer the possibility of providing for the first time brain anatomic predictors of treatment response in patients with major depression.

In view of the high prevalence of structural brain abnormalities seen in our depressed ECT population, it will be important to examine their impact on the therapeutic and adverse cognitive effects of ECT. Although anecdotal reports and small retrospective studies have suggested that depressed patients with organic brain disease may show a good clinical response to ECT without major adverse effects on cognitive functioning (Price and McAllister 1989), our ongoing studies are the first prospective investigations to address this issue directly. Preliminary findings indicate that most patients with subcortical hyperintensity, cortical atrophy, and ventriculomegaly will show a good clinical response to ECT, although some may experience an increased severity of cognitive side effects. More work is needed, however, to determine the precise relationship between particular structural brain abnormalities and clinical outcome, not only from ECT but from drug therapy as well. Finally, the impact of structural brain abnormalities on the long-term prognosis of the depressed elderly needs to be investigated. At least some elderly patients with depression appear to have a relatively poor outcome (Murphy 1983; Post 1972), and ventricular enlargement on CT has been found to be associated with a higher 2-year mortality in one study of elderly depressed subjects (Jacoby and Levy 1980). Long-term follow-up investigations are under way in one laboratory to determine the prognosis of depressed patients with structural brain disease.

In summary, the brains of elderly depressed subjects referred for ECT exhibit a variety of structural brain abnormalities, including cortical atrophy, subcortical hyperintensity, and lateral ventricular enlargement. Our preliminary data suggest that the presence of structural brain abnormalities may have important implications for the clinical phenomenology, biological markers, treatment, prognosis, and possibly pathophysiology of depressive illness in the elderly. Work is currently under way using more quantitative MRI measurement techniques to define in greater detail the extent and regional specificity of these abnormalities and their relationship to psychopathology in the elderly.

REFERENCES

American Psychiatric Association: Diagnostic and Statistical Manual of Mental Disorders, 3rd Edition. Washington, DC, American Psychiatric Association, 1980

Baxter LR, Phelps ME, Mazziotta JC, et al: Cerebral metabolic rates for glucose in mood disorders. Arch Gen Psychiatry 42:441–447, 1985

Caplan LR, Schmahmann JD, Baquis CD, et al: Caudate infarcts. Neurology 38(suppl):262, 1988

Coffey CE, Figiel GS: Neuropsychiatric significance of subcortical encephalomalacia, in Psychopathology and the Brain. Edited by Carroll BJ. New York, Raven (in press)

Coffey CE, Hinkle PE, Weiner RD, et al: Electroconvulsive therapy of depression in patients with white matter hyperintensity. Biol Psychiatry 22:626–629, 1987

Coffey CE, Figiel GS, Djang WT, et al: Effects of ECT upon brain structure: a pilot prospective magnetic resonance imaging study. Am J Psychiatry 145:701–706, 1988a

Coffey CE, Figiel GS, Djang WT, et al: Leukoencephalopathy in elderly depressed patients referred for ECT. Biol Psychiatry 24:143–161, 1988b

Coffey CE, Figiel GS, Djang WT, et al: Subcortical white matter hyperintensity on magnetic resonance imaging: clinical and neuroanatomic correlates in the depressed elderly. Journal of Neuropsychiatry 1:135–144, 1989

Coffey CE, Figiel GS, Djang WT, et al: Subcortical hyperintensity on magnetic resonance imaging: a comparison of normal and depressed elderly subjects. Am J Psychiatry 145:187–189, 1990

Dolan RJ, Calloway SP, Mann AH: Cerebral ventricular size in depressed subjects. Psychol Med 15:873–878, 1985

Dolan RJ, Calloway SP, Thacker PF, et al: The cerebral cortical appearance in depressed subjects. Psychol Med 16:775–779, 1986

Dorzab J, Baker M, Winokur G, et al: Depressive disease: clinical course. Diseases of the Nervous System 32:269–273, 1971

Drayer BP, Heyman A, Wilkinson W, et al: Early-onset Alzheimer's disease: an analysis of CT findings. Ann Neurol 17:407–410, 1985

Dupont RM, Jernigan TL, Butlers N, et al: Subcortical abnormalities in bipolar affective disorder using MRI. Arch Gen Psychiatry 47:55–59, 1990

Fazekas F, Chawluk JB, Alavi A, et al: MR signal abnormalities at 1.5T in Alzheimer's dementia and normal aging. American Journal of Neuroradiology 8:416–421, 1987

Figiel GS, Coffey CE, Weiner RD: Brain magnetic resonance imaging in elderly depressed patients receiving electroconvulsive therapy. Convulsive Therapy 5:26–34, 1989

Figiel GS, Coffey CE, Djang WT, et al: Brain MRI correlates of ECT-induced delirium. Journal of Neuropsychiatry and Clinical Neurosciences 2:53–58, 1990

George AE, deLeon MJ, Kalvin A, et al: Leukoencephalopathy in normal and pathologic aging. American Journal of Neuroradiology 7:567–570, 1986

Guy W (ed): ECDEU Assessment Manual for Psychopharmacology (Publ No ADM 76-338). Rockville, MD, U.S. Department of Health, Education and Welfare, 1976

Jacoby RJ, Levy R: Computed tomography in the elderly: affective disorder. Br J Psychiatry 136:270–275, 1980

Jacoby RJ, Dolan RJ, Levy R, et al: Quantitative computed tomography in elderly depressed patients. Br J Psychiatry 143:124–127, 1983

Jeste DV, Cullum M, Jernigan T, et al: Late-onset schizophrenia: neurophysiology and MRI. Paper presented at the annual meeting of the American Psychiatric Association, Montreal, Quebec, Canada, May 10, 1988a

Jeste DV, Lohr JB, Goodwin FK: Neuroanatomical studies of major affective disorders. Br J Psychiatry 153:444–459, 1988b

Kelsoe JR, Cadet JL, Pickar D, et al: Quantitative neuroanatomy in schizophrenia. Arch Gen Psychiatry 45:533–541, 1988

Kolbeinsson H, Arnaldsson OS, Peturrson H, et al: Computed tomographic scans in ECT patients. Acta Psychiatr Scand 73:28–32, 1986

Krishnan KRR, Goli V, Ellinwood EH, et al: Leukoencephalopathy in patients diagnosed as major depression. Biol Psychiatry 23:519–522, 1988

Largen JW Jr, Smith RC, Calderon M, et al: Abnormalities of brain structure and density in schizophrenia. Biol Psychiatry 19:991–1013, 1984

Miller BL, Lesser IM, Boone K, et al: Brain white-matter lesions and psychosis. Br J Psychiatry 155:73–78, 1989

Mori E, Yamadori A: Acute confusional state and acute agitated delirium. Arch Neurol 44:1139–1143, 1987

Murphy E: The prognosis of depression in old age. Br J Psychiatry 142:111–119, 1983

Nasrallah HA, Coffman HA, Olson SC: Structural brain imaging findings in affective disorders: an overview. Journal of Neuropsychiatry and Clinical Neurosciences 1:21–26, 1989

Pearlson GD, Wang DF, Ross C, et al: High DA D_2 receptors in psychotic bipolars on PET. Paper presented at the annual meeting of the American Psychiatric Association, Montreal, Quebec, Canada, May 11, 1988

Post F: The management and nature of depressive illnesses in late life: a follow-through study. Br J Psychiatry 121:393–404, 1972

Price TRP, McAllister TW: Safety and efficacy of ECT in depressed patients with dementia: a review of clinical experience. Convulsive Therapy 5:61–74, 1989

Rossi A, Stratt P, Petruzzi C, et al: A computerized tomographic study in DSM-III affective disorders. J Affective Disord 12:259–262, 1987

Rothschild AJ, Benes F, Woods B, et al: Cortisol and brain CT relationships in depression. Paper presented at the annual meeting of the American Psychiatric Association, Montreal, Quebec, Canada, May 9, 1988

Schatzberg AF, Rothschild AJ, Langlais PJ, et al: Cortisol, dopamine and psychosis in depression. Paper presented at the annual meeting of the American Psychiatric Association, Montreal, Quebec, Canada, May 11, 1988

Seab JP, Jagust WJ, Want STS, et al: Quantitative NMR measurements of hippocampal atrophy in Alzheimer's disease. Magn Reson Med 8:200–208, 1988

Shima S, Shikano T, Kitamura T, et al: Depression and ventricular enlargement. Acta Psychiatr Scand 70:275–277, 1984

Siegel JM: Brainstem mechanisms generating REM sleep, in Principles and Practice of Sleep. Edited by Kryger MH, Roth TC. Philadelphia, PA, WB Saunders, 1989, pp 104–120

Suddath RL, Casanova MF, Goldberg TE, et al: Temporal lobe pathology in schizophrenia: a quantitative magnetic resonance imaging study. Am J Psychiatry 146:464–472, 1989

Yates WR, Jacoby CG, Andreasen NC: Cerebellar atrophy in schizophrenia and affective disorder. Am J Psychiatry 144:465–467, 1987

Chapter 5

Neuroimaging in Secondary Affective Disorders

Joseph B. Bryer, M.D., Sergio E. Starkstein, M.D., Helen S. Mayberg, M.D., Robert G. Robinson, M.D.

During the past decade, the use of neuroimaging has provided valuable information about the structural brain abnormalities that may play a role in the etiology or mechanism of primary affective disorder. The neuroimaging techniques that have been particularly useful for identifying structural abnormalities in affective disorder as well as other psychiatric conditions include computed tomography (CT) and magnetic resonance imaging (MRI). Positron-emission tomography (PET), single photon emission computed tomography (SPECT), and xenon inhalation scans have been useful for identifying abnormalities in neuroreceptors, blood flow, and metabolic activity. Many of these studies are described in other chapters of this text.

One of the major problems in using neuroimaging to study primary affective disorders, however, is that the neuropathology that is etiologically related to this condition remains unknown (hence the term *primary affective disorder*). On the other hand, neuroimaging techniques are particularly well suited to identify the location and size of structural lesions in the living brain. We have tried to capitalize on this imaging capability by studying affective disorder in patients with structural brain lesions. The most readily available patients with focal injuries are those with strokes. They are the subjects of most of the studies we will describe in this chapter.

We have used a technique (i.e., the clinical-pathologic correlation following a spontaneous brain lesion) that was utilized by Broca as

---

The authors are greatly indebted to Drs. Thomas R. Price, John R. Lipsey, Marcelo Berthier, Godfrey D. Pearlson, Paul Fedoroff, Rajesh M. Parikh, and Karen Bolla-Wilson and Mrs. Paula Andrzejewski, who participated in many of these studies. This work was supported by the following National Institutes of Health grants: Research Scientist Award MH00163 (R.G.R.), MH40355, MH15178, NS15080 (H.S.M.), MH15330 (J.B.B.), and a grant from the University of Buenos Aires (S.E.S.).

far back as the 1860s to identify brain regions that play an important role in specific behaviors (Broca 1861). Three main neuroimaging approaches have been employed. First, we have correlated aspects of the stroke lesion visualized by CT or MRI, such as location and size, with the occurrence of affective disorders. Second, morphological analysis of the ventricular system of the brain using CT has been correlated with clinical presentation to try to identify premorbid neuropathologic risk factors for mood disorders following stroke. Finally, PET has been correlated with clinical findings to look for changes in monoamine neuroreceptor binding associated with the presence or development of depression.

IMAGING TECHNIQUES

Before discussing our findings in greater detail, it may be useful to discuss briefly the strengths and weaknesses of each of the imaging techniques that we have utilized. Most investigations into the relationship between lesion location and clinical presentation have utilized CT scans without contrast enhancement. Advantages of the noncontrast scan technique are that scans are usually easy to obtain, entail no risk to stroke patients, and are effective in demonstrating most stroke lesions of at least moderate size within 7–10 days of the lesion.

The main disadvantages of this technique are that CT may fail to reveal small lesions (particularly during the first 2–3 days after stroke) and that lesions in the posterior fossa are often poorly visualized due to bony artifacts. Although the cost of MRI is usually greater than that of CT, MRI is more sensitive than CT in demonstrating small lesions, as well as posterior fossa and brain stem lesions. In addition, since resolution and gray-white matter differentiation are superior in MRI, this modality may allow a more accurate delineation of specific structures affected by a lesion. Furthermore, the fact that MRI does not use ionizing radiation allows investigators to perform repeated scans in the same patient. Not all stroke lesions, however, are visualized with MRI.

Studies utilizing radiolabeled compounds such as the positron-emitting ligand (3-*N*-[^{11}C]methyl)spiperone (NMSP) and PET imaging allow the visualization of chemically specific receptor binding in the living brain. The strength of this technique is that receptor anatomy can be visualized and quantified within discrete brain regions in vivo. Receptor density (Bmax) and affinity (Kd) for different ligands can be quantified using a variety of methods including multicompartmental modeling, kinetic analysis, competitive inhibition with specific receptor antagonist, and studies with high- and low-specific-activity tracers. These precise measurements are often estimated using the ratio of activity in receptor-rich regions to receptor-poor regions (specific/nonspecific binding). This method may be preferable in patients who can tolerate only a single study where the question involves the comparison of the lesion with the nonlesion hemisphere. Difficulties may arise in precisely identifying borders separating injured and noninjured brain areas within the same hemisphere. Measurements made in incorrectly identified "nonlesion" tissue will affect quantitation of receptor binding measurements in these brain regions due to altered blood flow (and therefore delivery of tracer) and partial volume effects. These factors may influence receptor binding in ways that are not related to neurotransmitter-mediated changes in receptor function or the clinical phenomenon being studied. In our studies, we have tried to deal with these problems by selecting brain regions that are distant from the CT scan visualized–lesion site for receptor analysis and by taking receptor measurements between 30 and 60 minutes after injection when a steady state has been reached and blood flow is no longer influencing ligand availability at the receptor site.

In summary, although there are limitations associated with each imaging method, techniques that allow both structural and functional examination of the living brain are available. The technique to be used depends on the goals of the study, but interpretation of findings must be evaluated in the light of the limitations inherent to that technique.

NEUROIMAGING IN POSTSTROKE DEPRESSION

Background

Although physicians have long recognized that patients with cerebrovascular disease are prone to depression (e.g., Bleuler 1953; Kraepelin 1921), many considered these depressions to be an understandable psychological reaction to the impairment or disability resulting from the stroke (e.g., Fisher 1961). More recently, however, several investigators have begun to study this issue systematically and have provided data suggesting that this is not the case. Folstein et al. (1977), for example, found significantly more depression among stroke patients compared with orthopedic patients matched for degree of disability. Finklestein et al. (1982) also found significantly more depressive symptoms in stroke patients compared with patients with other medical illnesses that required rehabilitation therapy. These findings, which were confirmed by numerous other investigations (e.g., Robinson et al. 1983; Robinson et al. 1984b; Sinyor et al. 1986), suggest that disability alone is not responsible for the incidence of depression among stroke patients and that depression may be a specific consequence of stroke.

Prevalence of Depression Following Stroke

A number of studies have examined the prevalence of depression among patients with recent stroke. In a study of 103 patients hospitalized for acute stroke, we found that 27% met modified DSM-III (American Psychiatric Association 1980) criteria for major depression and 20% met modified DSM-III criteria for dysthymic (minor) depression (Robinson et al. 1983). Ebrahim et al. (1987) reported a prevalence of severe depression of 23% and of mild-moderate depression of 23% among acute stroke patients admitted to a general hospital. Sinyor et al. (1986) studied a consecutive series of stroke patients admitted to a rehabilitation hospital and found prevalences for mild, moderate, and severe depression of 17%, 23%, and 9%, respectively. Using Research Diagnostic Criteria (Spitzer et al. 1978), Eastwood et al. (1989), found that 10% of 87 patients admitted to a rehabilitation hospital met criteria for major depression; 40% met criteria for minor depression. In summary, all of the existing studies of depressive disorders following stroke have consistently found that depression is a frequent consequence, occurring in 30% to 50% of patients.

CT Scan Analysis of Lesions

Before beginning an analysis of lesion size or location, important basic variables that can influence CT imaging, such as the absence of head tilting and artifacts (e.g., metal objects, shunts) and consistency of slice thickness and angle to the canthomeatal line, must be determined. Each slice can then be examined for the presence of vascular lesions, and the area involved localized based on the anatomic correspondence between the damaged area and the homologous area in the Matsui and Hirano (1978) atlas. Using the method described by Levine and Grek (1984), the areas involved are grouped into the following regions: 1) central gyri (precentral and/or postcentral), 2) superior frontal gyrus, 3) frontotemporal (opercular) region (middle frontal gyrus, inferior frontal gyrus, insula and anterior temporal tip), 4) basal temporo-occipital region (inferior temporal gyrus, fusiform gyrus, hippocampal gyrus, lingual gyrus, cuneus), 5) temporoparietal region (superior temporal gyrus, middle temporal gyrus, supramarginal gyrus, angular gyrus), 6) superior parietal lobe, 7) occipital convexity, 8) lenticular nucleus, 9) caudate nucleus, 10) thalamus, 11) anterior limb of the internal capsule, 12) posterior limb of the internal capsule, and 13) corona radiata.

Lesions are then transferred onto templates (i.e., schematic brain drawings) by matching the CT slice with the corresponding template and drawing the lesion based on whether specific cortical gyri and/or subcortical structures are involved.

Mazzocchi and Vignolo (1978) described a method to localize cortical lesions (as visualized by CT) in the saggital plane. This method involves first identifying the angle of the CT sections from the orbitomeatal line by noting the presence or absence of specific landmark structures, such as the orbital roof, the sella turcica, and cerebrospinal fluid (CSF) spaces. Lines parallel to the real CT angle are traced, and the distance between the lines is kept proportional to the thickness of the slice. Then the contour of the lesion is traced in each slice and reconstructed on a saggital diagram.

These template methods are used to compare lesion locations from one patient to another and to determine if there are common structures that are associated with a particular clinical manifestation (e.g., depression). One example of the utility of this kind of CT scan analysis is a study in which we found that patients with depression following right hemisphere lesions had virtually no overlap in location of brain damage compared with patients with right hemisphere lesions and mania (Robinson et al. 1988a).

The size of the lesion can be determined using a computerized area calculation program and cursor pen. The area within the lesion is determined for each slice by tracing around the borders of the lesion and multiplying by the slice thickness. These volumes are then added together and divided by the volume of the whole brain. Whole-brain volume is determined by tracing the border of the whole brain (excluding ventricles) in nine dorsal slices beginning with the one that first includes frontal lobe tissue. An approximation to this value can be obtained by dividing the area of the largest cross section of the lesion by the area of the brain on the slice that passed through the body of the lateral ventricles.

The anterior-posterior location of the lesion is determined by measuring the distance in millimeters to the anterior and posterior borders of the lesion from the front of the brain and averaging over the slices where the lesion is visualized or alternatively using the single most proximal measurement (Figure 5-1).

In summary, CT scan analysis of lesions involves three elements. The first one is to construct a template in which multiple lesions are plotted on a schematic representation of the brain so that involved regions or structures that are common to a specific clinical presentation can be identified. The second element is to determine the volume of the lesion by using computerized semiautomated area calculation procedures. The third element is to measure quantitatively the borders of the lesion in the anterior-posterior dimension.

Relationship of Depression to Lesion Size and Location

Utilizing these CT scan analysis techniques, we have found that both interhemispheric lesion location and intrahemispheric lesion location are important in the production of poststroke mood disorders. In one study of 36 patients who had no previous history of brain injury or family or personal history of depression, patients with left hemisphere lesions had a higher, but not statistically significant, frequency of major depression (i.e., 7 of 22) than those with right hemisphere lesions (i.e., 2 of 14) (Robinson et al. 1984a). We also found, however, that severity of depression was related to the intrahemispheric lesion location, as described below.

We arbitrarily considered anterior lesions to be those for which the distance of the anterior border of the lesion to the frontal pole is less than 40% of the total anterior-posterior distance. Using this anterior-posterior distinction, we found that among patients with anterior lesions of the left hemisphere there was a significantly higher fre-

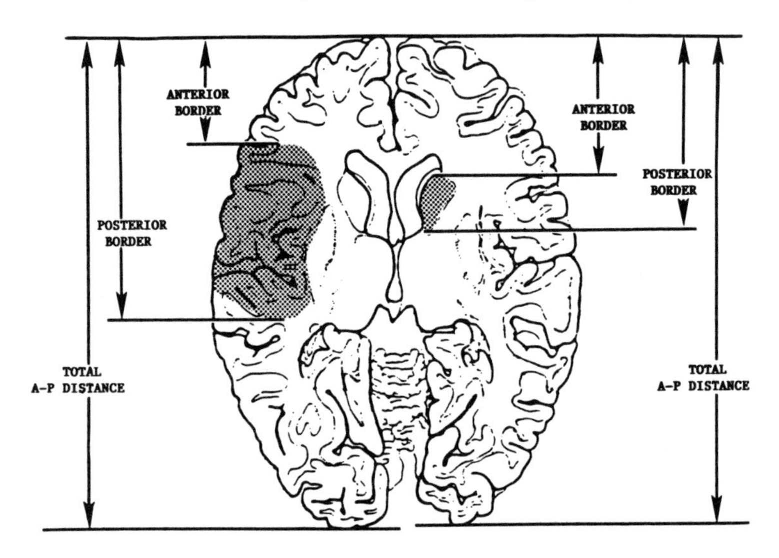

Figure 5-1. Schematic representation of a computed tomography image on which a cortical (*left*) and a subcortical (*right*) stroke lesion are represented (*shaded areas*). Anterior and posterior borders of the lesions are calculated as a percentage of the total anterior-posterior (A-P) distance of the affected hemisphere.

quency of major depression (i.e., 6 of 10) than among patients with lesions in any other location (i.e., 2 of 20) (χ^2 = 8.5, P < .01) (Robinson et al. 1984a). In addition to the left "anterior" lesion location being related to frequency of depression, the proximity of the anterior border of the lesion to the frontal pole was also found to correlate significantly with severity of depression (Robinson et al. 1984a). Among patients with left hemisphere lesions, the closer the lesion was to the frontal pole, the more severe the depression score. In contrast, among patients with right hemisphere lesions, higher depression scores were associated with more posterior lesions. Figure 5-2 illustrates these relationships of lesion location to severity of depression.

This relationship between left anterior lesion location and depression appears to hold equally well for both cortical and subcortical

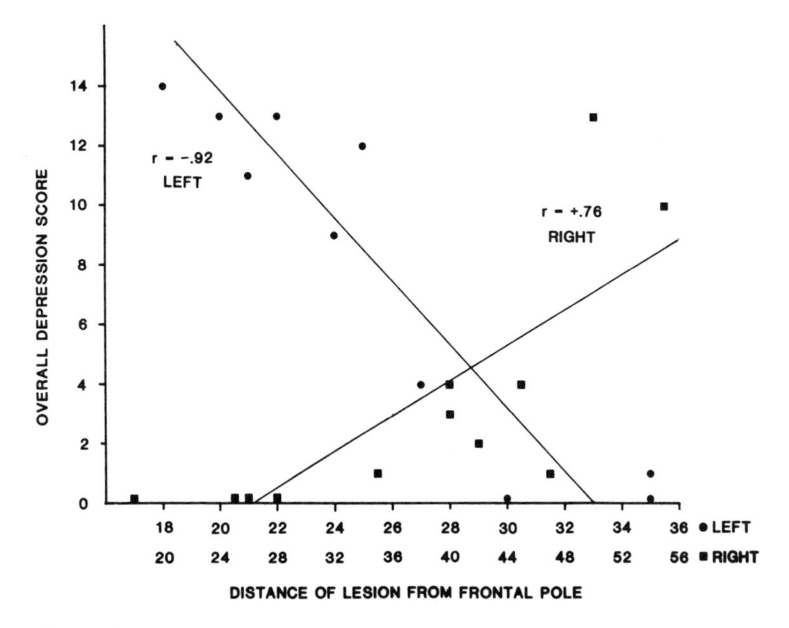

Figure 5-2. Relationship between overall depression score and distance of the anterior border of the lesion from the frontal pole for patients with either left anterior infarcts or right hemisphere infarcts. Distance is expressed as a percentage of the total anterior-posterior distance. Correlation coefficients are shown: left, r = −.92, P < .001; right, r = .76, P < .01. Reprinted from Robinson RG, Kubos KL, Starr LB, et al: Mood disorders in stroke patients: importance of location of lesion. Brain 107:81–93, 1984. By permission of Oxford University Press.

lesions. In a study subsequent to the one previously described, we found that the frequency of major depression among patients with left anterior subcortical lesions (4 of 6 patients) was significantly greater than among patients with left posterior subcortical lesions (0 of 7 patients) ($\chi^2 = 6.7$, $P < .01$) or patients with right subcortical lesions (1 of 7 patients) ($\chi^2 = 3.7$, $P < .05$) (Starkstein et al. 1987a). Among those with cortical lesions of the left hemisphere, the frequency of major depression was 3 of 5 in patients with anterior lesions and 1 of 11 for those with posterior lesions ($\chi^2 = 6.7$, $P < .01$). In addition, there was a statistically significant correlation between the severity of depression as measured by score on the Present State Exam (Wing et al. 1974) and by the distance of the lesion from the frontal pole for both cortical and subcortical lesions (Figure 5-3).

The strong association between left anterior lesion location and depression has also been found in patients with bilateral infarcts. Lipsey et al. (1983) reported that patients whose multiple lesions included a left anterior lesion were significantly more depressed than patients with multiple lesions but without a left anterior infarct. Neither right hemisphere lesion location nor temporal sequence of the multiple lesions correlated significantly with severity of depression.

Although there have been only a few other investigators who have examined this issue of the relationship between depression and anterior-posterior lesion location, Eastwood et al. (1989) reported a significant correlation ($r = -.74$, $P < .05$) between severity of depression and proximity of the lesion to the frontal pole only for patients with left hemisphere lesions. A reanalysis of the Sinyor et al. (1986) data also reveals a significant correlation ($r = 0.47$, $P < .05$) between depression and proximity of the lesion to the frontal pole among patients with anterior lesions of either hemisphere (Robinson et al. 1988b).

Starkstein et al. (1988b) provided further evidence of a specific relationship between lesion location and major depression by comparing depressive disorders in 37 patients with posterior circulation (PC) strokes to those in 42 patients with middle cerebral artery (MCA) infarcts. Patients with brain stem or cerebellar infarcts had a significantly lower frequency of depression (4 of 37 with major, 6 of 37 with minor) than those with MCA territory lesions (11 of 42 with major, 9 of 42 with minor) ($\chi^2 = 3.54$, $P = .05$). Furthermore, those with PC infarcts who were depressed recovered from depression more quickly than depressed patients with MCA territory lesions; that is, at 6-month follow-up, 82% of the MCA patients with inhospital depression were still depressed, whereas only 20% of the PC patients with

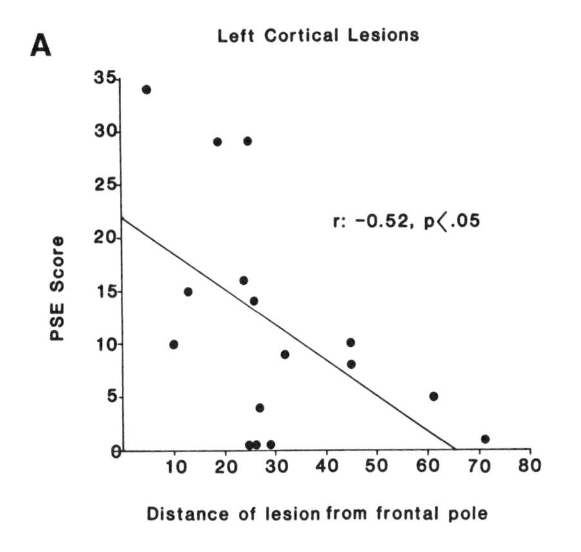

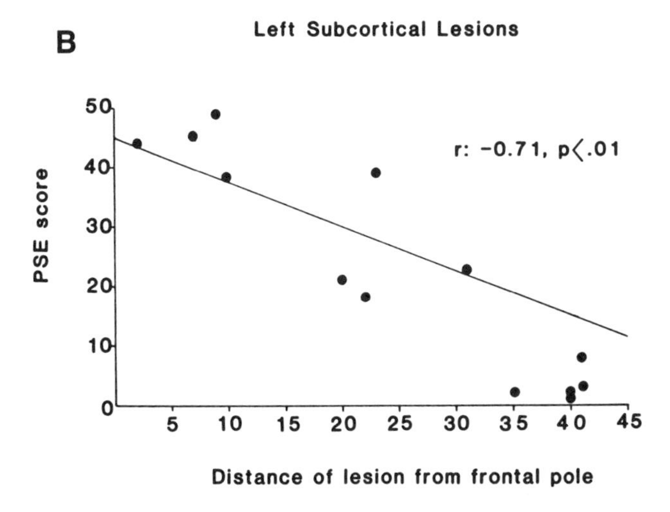

Figure 5-3. Relationship between Present State Exam (PSE) score and distance of the anterior border of the lesion from the frontal pole for patients with left cortical (*A*) and left subcortical (*B*) lesions. Distance is expressed as a percentage of the total anterior-posterior distance. Reprinted from Starkstein SE, Robinson RG, Price TR: Comparison of cortical and subcortical lesions in the production of post-stroke mood disorders. Brain 110:1045–1059, 1987. By permission of Oxford University Press.

inhospital depression remained depressed, ($\chi^2 = 3.7$, $P < .05$). On the basis of these findings, we have suggested that poststroke depression following lesions in different brain areas may have different mechanisms.

The association between lesion volume and depression appears to be a relatively minor one, compared to the importance of lesion location. In the study of 36 patients previously described (Robinson et al. 1984a), among patients with left anterior lesions, lesion volume (the mean was 4.7% of total brain volume in this group) correlated significantly with severity of depression. No such correlation, however, was observed among patients with left posterior, right anterior, or right posterior lesions. Although significant correlations between depression and lesion volume have not been found in all studies (Robinson and Szetela 1981; Starkstein et al. 1987a), some subsequent studies have confirmed a weak correlation between lesion volume and severity of depression (Eastwood et al. 1989).

In addition to the strong relationship between depression and *intra*hemispheric lesion location, there also appears to be a relationship between depression and *inter*hemispheric lesion location. Although there is quite a bit of evidence that there are interhemispheric asymmetries in the processing of emotion and response to injury (Borod et al. 1985; Gainotti 1972; Tucker 1980), some investigators have reported increased prevalence of depression among those with left hemisphere injury (deBonis et al. 1985; Finklestein et al. 1982), whereas others have not (Dam et al. 1989; Eastwood et al. 1989; Folstein et al. 1977; Sinyor et al. 1986).

Why hemispheric side of the lesion sometimes seems to be related to frequency of depression and sometimes does not is an interesting issue. We believe the answer to this problem is that interhemispheric lesion location is only one of many factors that can influence the expression of affective disorder following stroke. For example, in a study of 93 patients with single lesions of the right hemisphere, we found that major depression was significantly more frequent following lesions of the parietal and dorsal lateral frontal cortex than any other location within the right hemisphere (Starkstein et al. 1989). In addition to these CT scan–identified lesion locations, however, major depression was found to be significantly more frequently associated with a family history of psychiatric disorder (5 of 17) compared with patients with other diagnoses following right hemisphere lesions (5 of 26) ($\chi^2 = 7.5$, $P < .01$) or with patients with major depression following left hemisphere lesions (1 of 27) ($\chi^2 = 4.4$, $P < .05$). These findings suggest that, in contrast to the patients with left hemisphere injury and major depression, some patients with right hemisphere injury and major depression have a genetic predisposition and therefore perhaps a different etiologic mechanism for their disorder.

Although it is not surprising that there may be multiple etiologies for major depression following stroke, it does emphasize the point that factors that can influence or cause depression following stroke must be controlled before the effect of a single variable like interhemispheric lesion location can be examined. Time since injury, diagnostic criteria, personal or family history of affective disorder, previous stoke, intrahemispheric lesion location, and subcortical atrophy (this will be discussed later) can all influence the affective response to stroke. In the section on neuroreceptor imaging, we will discuss one possible explanation for this phenomenon of interhemispheric differences in emotional response to stroke.

In summary, neuroimaging of lesion size and location has led to a number of intriguing clinical-pathologic correlations in poststroke depression. The use of templates for localization of lesions has identified that left frontal cortex and left basal ganglia injury are strongly associated with major depressive disorders. In addition, for both cortical and subcortical lesions, there is a significant correlation between the proximity of the lesion to the frontal pole and severity of depression. Interhemispheric lesion location also seems to play a role in depressive disorders, with left hemisphere lesions more likely to lead to depression when a large number of factors that may lead to etiologically different conditions are controlled.

Major Depression Versus Minor Depression

Neuroimaging techniques have also been useful in validating the distinction between the two types of depressive disorders that we have identified (i.e., major depression and minor depression). As indicated previously, the diagnoses of major depression and minor depression are based on the symptoms (but not duration) criteria of DSM-III for dysthymic disorder or major depression. These symptoms are elicited by use of the Present State Exam, a semistructured psychiatric interview.

Three lines of evidence suggest that poststroke minor depression is not simply a less severe form of major depression, but instead represents a distinct type of affective disorder (Starkstein and Robinson 1989). First, major depression in stroke patients usually spontaneously remits within 1 to 2 years, whereas minor depression runs a chronic course, usually greater than 2 years (Robinson et al. 1984c; Robinson et al. 1987). Second, major depression but not minor depression is associated with both a dementia of depression ("pseudodementia") and nonsuppression of serum cortisol following dexamethasone administration (Bolla-Wilson et al. 1989; Lipsey et al. 1985; Robinson et al. 1986). Third, neuroimaging studies have demonstrated that only major depression is significantly associated with left frontal and left basal ganglia lesions. In contrast, minor depression is significantly associated with right parietal and dorsal lateral frontal lobe lesions (Starkstein et al. 1989). These findings suggest that stroke may lead to at least two phenomenologically distinct forms of mood disorder and that these mood disorders may be provoked by different pathologic mechanisms.

POSTSTROKE MANIA

Mania is another form of mood disorder that has been reported to follow stroke and therefore is potentially accessible to study using neuroimaging. Because of the low frequency of secondary mania among stroke patients, however, the psychiatric literature has been dominated by anecdotal reports on this disorder. We have, however, studied 17 patients with secondary mania: 9 had stroke, 6 had tumors, and 2 had traumatic brain injury (Robinson et al. 1988a). Of the 9 stroke patients, 8 sustained a right unilateral lesion. The right hemisphere structures involved were the head of the caudate nucleus, thalamus, basotemporal cortex, and orbitofrontal cortex. In contrast to our findings among patients with depression, however, there was no significant correlation between proximity of the lesion to the frontal pole and severity or frequency of mania. These findings were in agreement with the suggestion of Cummings and Mendez (1984) that damage to right hemispheric limbic structures (or limbic-connected structures) is necessary for the production of poststroke mania. In addition to the association with lesion location, a family history of affective disorder was present in 4 of the 9 stroke patients and was significantly more frequent than among patients with poststroke major depression (i.e., 3 of 31) ($\chi^2 = 4.1$, $P < .05$) (Robinson et al. 1988a).

In summary, our studies of mania following brain injury have utilized the same neuroimaging techniques for clinical-pathologic correlation as we used for depressive disorders. In contrast to depressive disorders, however, mania is associated with right hemisphere lesions in limbic-connected areas of the brain, including the orbitofrontal cortex, basotemporal cortex, basal ganglia, and thalamus. A family history of affective disorder and subcortical atrophy (as will be discussed next) appear to be premorbid risk factors for the development of mania following a right hemisphere lesion.

SUBCORTICAL ATROPHY IN POSTSTROKE MOOD DISORDERS

Previous discussion of our findings using neuroimaging techniques has focused on the lesion itself and clinical-pathologic correlations that can be made using template reconstructions and measurements of lesion size and location. Another neuroimaging technique that has been useful in studying a variety of psychiatric disorders is measurement of ventricular brain ratios (VBRs). VBRs and measurement of cortical "sulci" width are quantitative measures of subcortical and cortical atrophy, respectively. They involve both linear and planimetric measurements of the third and lateral ventricles and surrounding landmarks, as well as cortical sulci. Although investigators still debate the relative utility of one measurement compared with another or planimetric compared with linear measures (Schlegel and Kretzschmar 1987), there are standardized methods that have been established for making these measurements (Gomori et al. 1984).

In an attempt to elucidate nonlesion factors that may explain why all patients with left frontal cortex or left basal ganglia lesions do not develop depression, we examined 13 pairs of patients matched for size and location of lesion, as well as time since brain injury (Starkstein et al. 1988a). One of each pair had poststroke major depression while the other was nondepressed. There were no significant differences between depressed and nondepressed patients in terms of neurologic impairments, social functioning, family or personal history of psychiatric disorders, or activities of daily living. Morphological analysis of the ventricular system, however, revealed significant between-group differences. We will briefly describe the methodology we used to measure cortical and subcortical atrophy.

The bifrontal ratio is the distance between the tips of the frontal horns divided by the distance between the inner tables of the skull along the same line. The bicaudate ratio is the minimal distance between the caudate indentations of the frontal horns divided by the distance between the inner tables of the skull along the same line. The third VBR is the multiple of the maximal sagittal and coronal diameters of the third ventricle divided by the multiple of the trans-pineal and the midsagittal inner diameters. The VBR was calculated as a planimetric measurement. The ventricular area was assessed at the level of the ventricular body, and the brain area was also measured at the same level. For this measurement, only the ventricle contralateral to the lesion location was assessed.

There are two measurements of cortical atrophy. *Frontal fissure ratio* is the maximal width of the interhemispheric fissure at the frontal level divided by the trans-pineal coronal inner table diameter. *Four cortical sulci ratio* is the sum of the widths of the four widest cortical sulci divided by the trans-pineal coronal inner table diameter.

Depressed patients had significantly higher mean third VBRs and lateral VBRs than the nondepressed matched controls. Of the 13 depressed patients, 10 had higher lateral VBRs than their matched controls. None of the cortical sulci ratios were significantly different between the depressed and nondepressed groups. Since CT scans were obtained in the immediate poststroke period and postinjury atrophy takes some time to develop, the increased VBR and third VBR were probably present prior to the stroke. Thus subcortical atrophy as evidenced by increased third VBR and VBR (with no cortical atrophy) may represent a risk factor for major depression following stroke.

We also examined this same issue in patients with poststroke mania. We compared 11 patients who developed mania after brain injury with 11 patients matched for age, time since injury, and size, location, and etiology of lesion (Starkstein et al. 1987b). Although the two groups were not significantly different in background characteristics, past personal history, or medications being taken at the time they developed mania, the secondary mania group had significantly larger third VBRs and bifrontal ratios. Between-group differences in the VBR were in the same direction but did not reach statistical significance. Thus, our findings suggest that subcortical atrophy may be an important risk factor for the development of mania as well as depression following stroke.

A number of other investigators have also reported evidence of subcortical atrophy among patients with "idiopathic" major depression or bipolar disorder (e.g., Pearlson and Veroff 1981; Scott et al. 1983). Although such findings are by no means specific for affective disorder, they do suggest that there may be neuropathologic similarities between idiopathic and poststroke mood disorders and that subcortical atrophy may play a permissive role in the development of these disorders.

In summary, the measurement of brain morphology based on neuroimaging is another variable that can be examined in secondary affective disorders. In studies where the effect of the lesion is eliminated (by matching patients for lesion size and location), we have found that mania (usually associated with right hemisphere lesions) and major depression (usually associated with left hemisphere lesions) are both associated with subcortical atrophy as evidenced by enlarged VBRs. The cause of this subcortical atrophy as well as its histologic pathology have yet to be determined, but this atrophy, which appears to play a permissive role in a variety of psychiatric disorders, is a risk factor for both mania and depression following stroke.

NEURORECEPTOR IMAGING IN POSTSTROKE MOOD DISORDERS

We have tried to illustrate how structural neuroimaging techniques have been useful in identifying important neuropathologic relationships in poststroke affective disorders. This kind of neuroimaging, however, has provided little information about alterations in function that result from stroke and that may be responsible for the signs and symptoms of mood disorder. The development of functional imaging techniques, including PET and SPECT, has provided investigators with powerful tools to address some of these important issues.

In light of substantial evidence implicating alterations in monoamine systems as one of the etiologic factors in affective disorder, we have investigated serotonin receptor binding using PET in poststroke depression (Mayberg et al. 1988). Seventeen patients with single stroke lesions of the right or left hemisphere were compared with 17 control subjects using the ligand NMSP. Although NMSP binds to both serotonin S_2 and dopamine D_2 receptors, there are few cortical dopamine receptors outside the prefrontal and cingulate cortex. Thus, cortical binding of NMSP primarily labels S_2 receptors (Mayberg et al. 1990). The patients were scanned an average of 16 months after stroke and underwent psychiatric interview and neurologic examination on the day of the scan. Eight patients had left hemisphere strokes, and 9 had right hemisphere strokes. Left and right hemisphere stroke groups did not differ significantly in terms of age, activities of daily living, lesion location or size, or cognitive impairment. Three of the patients with right hemisphere stroke and one with a left hemisphere stroke met criteria for major depression; one patient with a left hemisphere stroke met criteria for minor depression. Neither mean depression scores nor frequency of diagnosis of depression differed between these groups.

NMSP binding was quantified by comparing regional activity (average counts per pixel corrected for injected dose) in homologous cortical regions in the injured and noninjured hemispheres (i.e., stroke/nonstroke cortical binding ratio). Control subjects showed a binding ratio of 1.0 (i.e., equal binding in left and right hemispheres) in the frontal, parietal, and temporal cortex. Relative to control subjects and left hemisphere stroke patients, patients with right hemisphere strokes showed higher binding ratios of ipsilateral (i.e., right hemisphere) to contralateral (i.e., left hemisphere) binding in both temporal and parietal cortex (Figure 5-4). Only areas that were not involved in the lesion by CT scan analysis were compared.

NMSP binding ratios were not significantly different between patients with left hemisphere stroke and control subjects for any of the cortical regions. The elevated ipsilateral-to-contralateral binding ratio in the right hemisphere stroke group appeared to be due to increased binding in the ipsilateral (right) cortical areas rather than decreased binding in the contralateral (left) cortical areas. Figure 5-5 shows CT and PET scans of a patient with a right frontal white matter infarct that displays this phenomenon.

In addition to this finding of increased S_2 receptors following right but not left hemisphere stroke, ipsilateral-to-contralateral binding in temporal cortex was inversely correlated with severity of depression among patients with left hemisphere strokes. Lower binding ratios in left temporal cortex were associated with higher depression scale scores. No statistically significant correlations between cortical binding ratios and depression scores were found for patients with right hemisphere strokes.

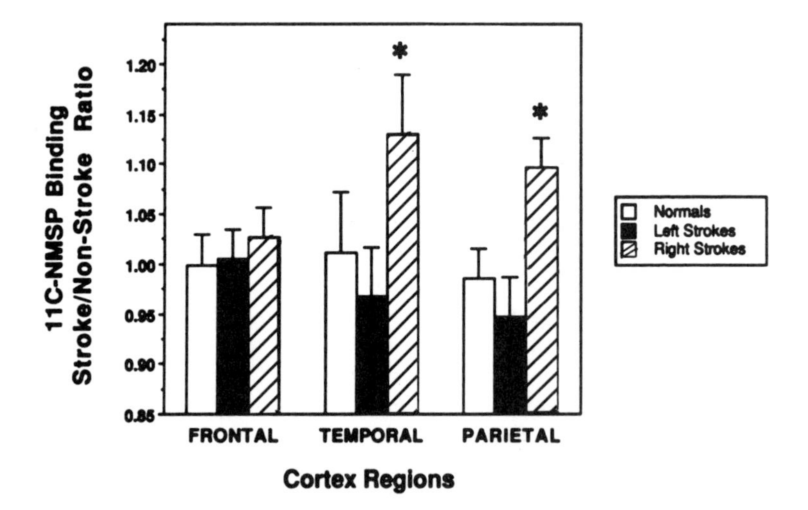

Figure 5-4. Ipsilateral-to-contralateral (3-*N*-[^{11}C]methyl)spiperone (NMSP) binding ratios in three cortical areas for patients with left (*solid bars*) or right (*hatched bars*) hemisphere stroke and for normal controls (*open bars*). Patients with right hemisphere lesions had significantly higher mean binding ratio in temporal and parietal cortex than normal controls or patients with left hemisphere injury. (Compared with normal controls, temporal: U = 116,37, 16 df, P = .018; parietal: U = 101,35, 16 df, P = .029.)

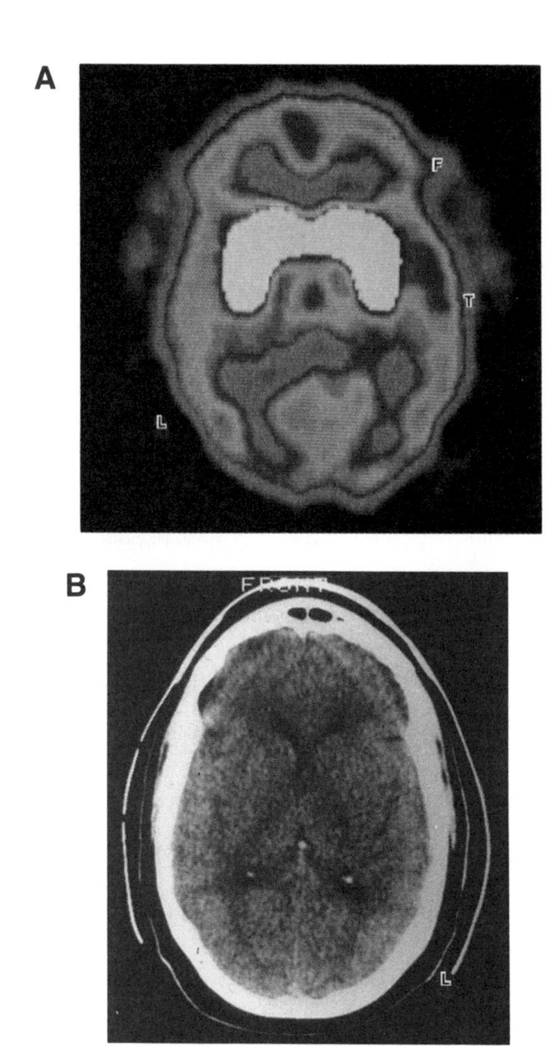

Figure 5-5. (3-*N*-[^{11}C]methyl)Spiperone binding (NMSP) (*A*) in a patient with a right hemisphere white matter infarct. The positron-emission tomography (PET) scan is at the level of (*B*) where the lesion is not visualized on computed tomography. The PET scan demonstrates the phenomenon of increased NMSP binding in the right temporal (*T*) cortical area relative to that area in left (*L*) hemisphere. *F* = frontal. Reprinted from Mayberg HS, Robinson RG, Wong DF, et al: PET imaging of cortical S_2 serotonin receptors after stroke: lateralized charges and relationship to depression. Am J Psychiatry 145:937–943, 1988. Copyright 1988. Reprinted by permission.

This study demonstrated for the first time a lateralized biochemical response following brain injury in humans. It is consistent both with previous studies showing a lateralized effect of stroke on neurotransmitter concentrations in rats (Robinson 1979) and with subsequent studies showing lateralized effects of brain injury on spiperone binding in rats (Mayberg et al. 1990). This binding is significant in light of much evidence that there are hemispheric asymmetries in the regulation of mood (Borod et al. 1985; Tucker 1980). It may represent a neurochemical basis for the clinical finding of a differential risk for mood disorder, depending on which hemisphere is injured.

This PET study also provided evidence that alterations in the serotonergic system may be etiologically associated with major depression, at least among patients with left hemisphere strokes. We also have preliminary findings of a significant reduction of the serotonin metabolite 5-hydroxyindoleacetic acid (5-HIAA) in the CSF of depressed acute stroke patients relative to nondepressed acute stroke patients.

MECHANISM OF POSTSTROKE DEPRESSION

Although the mechanism by which stroke lesions lead to the development of depression remains unknown, the PET and other findings suggest that one possible mechanism of poststroke major depression may be related to reduced serotonergic neurotransmission. Ascending noradrenergic and serotonergic axons originate in cell bodies in the brain stem, ascend anteriorly in the median forebrain bundle, and pass through the striatum and into the frontal cortex. Some fibers terminate in the frontal cortex while most fibers arc posteriorly over the genu of the corpus callosum and run anteriorly to posteriorly through the deep layers of the cortex with arborizations to more superficial layers in all areas of cortex (Morrison et al. 1979). Given this anatomy, depression following acute stroke may be related to reduced serotonin release, with anterior lesions affecting monoamine innervation of larger areas of cortex than more posterior lesions. Chronic poststroke major depression among patients with left hemisphere stroke may be related to a failure to compensate for reduced serotonin release by up-regulating serotonin receptor density. Such a pathologic mechanism is not inconsistent with the action of various antidepressants and electroconvulsive therapy (e.g., Evans et al. 1976) and is supported by studies in rats that examined the effect of lesion location on monoamines (Pearlson et al. 1984) and the lateralized effect of cortical lesions on S_2 receptor binding (Mayberg et al. 1990).

SUMMARY AND DIRECTIONS FOR FUTURE RESEARCH

Although much remains unknown about affective disorders following brain injury, both structural and neuroreceptor imaging techniques have been valuable tools in advancing understanding of the etiology and mechanism of these disorders. In this chapter, we have reviewed the strengths and weaknesses of each imaging technique and emphasized that clinical-pathologic correlations based on each technique must be interpreted with the limitations of that imaging method in mind. For example, measurement of the boundaries of a lesion or its area depends on when the scan was done after injury, how much edema occurred, whether intraparenchymal bleeding occurred, and so on. We have discussed how we use template construction, volume measurements, and lesion border measurements to analyze and correlate clinical presentation with lesion variables.

Using these methods, our most important findings from neuroimaging analysis are that major depression is significantly more likely to occur after left frontal cortical and left basal ganglia lesions than after lesion to any other location. Mania, on the other hand, is significantly more likely to occur following right orbitofrontal or basotemporal cortical lesions or right basal ganglia or thalamic lesions.

In addition to lesion analysis, we have shown how morphological analysis of the ventricular system of the brain can also be a useful technique for studying secondary affective disorders. When the effect of lesion location is controlled, subcortical atrophy (i.e., enlarged VBRs without widening of cortical sulci) appears to play a permissive role and represents an important risk factor for both major depression and mania following brain injury.

Finally, we showed how functional brain imaging using PET can provide insights into the mechanism of secondary affective disorder that are not possible with structural imaging. Using NMSP to label cortical S_2 receptors, we found that patients with right hemisphere strokes had an increase in S_2 receptors in uninjured areas of the temporal and parietal cortex, whereas patients with left hemisphere stroke did not. The severity of depression, however, correlated with paucity of S_2 receptors in the left temporal cortex, suggesting that the lack of up-regulation of S_2 receptors after left hemisphere injury may explain why depression is associated with left frontal and left basal ganglia strokes.

There are numerous areas for future research using neuroimaging in secondary affective disorders. For example, the improved structural imaging available with MRI scanning may better define exactly which brain structures are most important in producing these affective syndromes. Since many small strokes are missed by CT, the improved imaging of MRI may also better define the clinical-pathologic relationships associated with these small lacunar strokes. Neuroimaging may also help to clarify the basis for differences from one patient to the next in clinical presentation. For example, in a recent study, we compared patients who had major depression with generalized anxiety disorder (approximately half of patients with major depression) to those without anxiety (Starkstein et al. 1990b). Analysis of lesion characteristics indicated that patients with anxiety had significantly greater frequency of cortical lesions, whereas depressed patients with no anxiety symptoms had a significantly greater frequency of subcortical lesions. Other variations in clinical presentation may also be illuminated by neuroimaging studies. Finally, there are many additional studies that could be done with PET imaging. We have conducted some preliminary metabolic studies in patients with secondary mania and found significant hypometabolic effects in the right basotemporal cortex, distant from the site of the lesion (Starkstein et al. 1990a). Thus, PET studies may help to define the mechanism by which a lesion leads to clinical symptoms. Further receptor studies may also define the biochemical mediators for these metabolic changes. Ultimately, the illumination of the mechanism of these secondary affective syndromes will allow the development of truly specific rational treatments for these disorders.

REFERENCES

American Psychiatric Association: Diagnostic and Statistical Manual of Mental Disorders, 3rd Edition. Washington, DC, American Psychiatric Association, 1980

Bleuler E: Textbook of Psychiatry. New York, Dover Publications, 1953

Bolla-Wilson K, Robinson RG, Starkstein SE, et al: Lateralization of dementia of depression in stroke patients. Am J Psychiatry 146:627–634, 1989

Borod JC, Koff E, Lorch MP: Channels of emotional expression in patients with unilateral brain damage. Arch Neurol 42:345–348, 1985

Broca P: A new finding of aphasia following a lesion of the posterior part of the second and third frontal convolutions. Bull de la Societe Anatomique 6:398–407, 1861

Cummings JL, Mendez MF: Secondary mania with focal cerebrovascular lesions. Am J Psychiatry 141:1084–1087, 1984

Dam H, Pederson HE, Ahlgren P: Depression among patients with stroke. Acta Psychiatr Scand 80:118–124, 1989 deBonis M, Dellatolas G, Rondot P: Mood disorders in left and right brain-damaged patients: comparison between ratings and self-ratings on the same adjective mood scale: some methodological problems. Psychopathology 18:286–292, 1985

Eastwood MR, Rifat SL, Nobbs H, et al: Mood disorder following cerebrovascular accident. Br J Psychiatry 154:195–200, 1989

Ebrahim S, Barer KD, Nouri P: Affective illness after stroke. Br J Psychiatry 151:52–56, 1987

Evans JP, Grahame-Smith DG, Green AR, et al: Electroconvulsive shock increases the behavioural responses of rats to brain 5-hydroxytryptamine accumulation and central nervous system stimulant drugs. Br J Pharmacol 56:193–199, 1976

Finklestein S, Benowitz LI, Baldessarini RG, et al: Mood, vegetative disturbance and dexamethasone suppression test after stroke. Ann Neurol 12:463–468, 1982

Fisher S: Psychiatric considerations of cerebral vascular disease. Am J Cardiol 7:379–385, 1961

Folstein MF, Maiberger R, McHugh PR: Mood disorder as a specific complication of stroke. J Neurol Neurosurg Psychiatry 40:1018–1020, 1977

Gainotti G: Emotional behavior and hemispheric side of lesion. Cortex 8:41–55, 1972

Gomori JM, Steiner I, Melamed E, et al: The assessment of changes in brain volume using combined linear measurements: a CT-scan study. Neuroradiology 26:21–24, 1984

Kraepelin E: Manic Depressive Insanity and Paranoia. Edinburgh, Livingstone, 1921

Levine DN, Grek A: The anatomic basis of delusions after right cerebral infarction. Neurology 34:577–582, 1984

Lipsey JR, Robinson RG, Pearlson GD, et al: Mood change following bilateral hemisphere brain injury. Br J Psychiatry 143:266–273, 1983

Lipsey JR, Robinson RG, Pearlson GD, et al: Dexamethasone suppression test and mood following stroke. Am J Psychiatry 142:318–323, 1985

Matsui T, Hirano H: An Atlas of the Human Brain for Computerized Tomography. New York, Igaku-Shoin Medical Publishers, 1978

Mayberg HS, Robinson RG, Wong DF, et al: PET imaging of cortical S_2 serotonin receptors after stroke: lateralized changes and relationship to depression. Am J Psychiatry 145:937–943, 1988

Mayberg HS, Moran TH, Robinson RG: Remote lateralized changes in cortical 3H-spiperone binding following focal frontal cortex lesions in the rat. Brain Res 516:127–131, 1990

Mazzocchi F, Vignolo LA: Computer assisted tomography in neuropsychological research: a simple procedure for lesion mapping. Cortex 14:136–144, 1978

Morrison JM, Molliver ME, Grzanna R: Noradrenergic innervation of cerebral cortex: widespread effects of local cortical lesions. Science 205:313–316, 1979

Pearlson GD, Veroff AF: Computerized tomographic scan changes in manic depressive illness. Lancet 2:470, 1981

Pearlson GD, Kubos KL, Robinson RG: Effect of anterior-posterior lesion locations on the asymmetrical behavioral and biochemical response to cortical suction ablations in the rat. Brain Res 293:241–250, 1984

Robinson RG: Differential behavioral and biochemical effects of right and left hemispheric cerebral infarction in the rat. Science 205:707–710, 1979

Robinson RG, Szetela B: Mood change following left hemispheric brain injury. Ann Neurol 9:447–453, 1981

Robinson RG, Starr LB, Kubos KL, et al: A two-year longitudinal study of post-stroke mood disorders: findings during the initial evaluation. Stroke 14:736–741, 1983

Robinson RG, Kubos KL, Starr LB, et al: Mood disorders in stroke patients: importance of location of lesion. Brain 107:81–93, 1984a

Robinson RG, Starr LB, Lipsey JR, et al: A two-year longitudinal study of post-stroke mood disorders: dynamic changes in associated variables over the first six months of follow-up. Stroke 15:510–517, 1984b

Robinson RG, Starr LB, Price TR: A two-year longitudinal study of post-stroke mood disorders: prevalence and duration at six months follow-up. Br J Psychiatry 144:256–262, 1984c

Robinson RG, Bolla-Wilson K, Kaplan E: Depression influences intellectual impairment in stroke patients. Br J Psychiatry 148:541–547, 1986

Robinson RG, Boldine PL, Price TR: Two-year longitudinal study of post-stroke mood disorders: diagnosis and outcome at one and two years. Stroke 18:837–843, 1987

Robinson RG, Boston JD, Starkstein SE, et al: Comparison of mania and depression after brain injury: causal factors. Am J Psychiatry 145:172–178, 1988a

Robinson RG, Starkstein SE, Price TR: Post-stroke depression and lesion location (letter). Stroke 19:125–126, 1988b

Schlegel S, Kretzschmar K: Computed tomography in affective disorders, Part I: ventricular and sulcal measurements. Biol Psychiatry 22:4–14, 1987

Scott ML, Golden CJ, Ruedrich SL: Ventricular enlargement in major depression. Psychiatry Res 8:91–93, 1983

Sinyor D, Jacques P, Kaloupek DG, et al: Post-stroke depression and lesion location: an attempted replication. Brain 109:537–546, 1986

Spitzer RL, Endicott J, Robins E: Research Diagnostic Criteria: rationale and reliability. Arch Gen Psychiatry 35:773–782, 1978

Starkstein SE, Robinson RG: Affective disorders and cerebrovascular disease. Br J Psychiatry 154:170–182, 1989

Starkstein SE, Robinson RG, Price TR: Comparison of cortical and subcortical lesions in the production of post-stroke mood disorders. Brain 110:1045–1059, 1987a

Starkstein SE, Pearlson GD, Boston JD, et al: Mania after brain injury: a controlled study of causative factors. Arch Neurol 44:1069–1073, 1987b

Starkstein SE, Robinson RG, Price TR: Comparison of patients with and without post-stroke major depression matched for size and location of lesion. Arch Gen Psychiatry 45:247–252, 1988a

Starkstein SE, Robinson RG, Berthier ML, et al: Depressive disorders following posterior circulation as compared with middle cerebral artery infarcts. Brain 11:375–387, 1988b

Starkstein SE, Robinson RG, Honig MA, et al: Mood changes after right hemisphere lesions. Br J Psychiatry 155:79–85, 1989

Starkstein SE, Mayberg HS, Berthier ML, et al: Mania after brain injury: neuroradiological and metabolic findings. Ann Neurol 27:652–659, 1990a

Starkstein SE, Cohen BS, Fedoroff P, et al: Relationship between anxiety disorders and depressive disorders in patients with cerebrovascular injury. Arch Gen Psychiatry 47:246–251, 1990b

Tucker DA: Lateral brain function, emotion and conceptualization. Psychol Bull 89:19–46, 1980

Wing JK, Cooper JE, Sartorius N: The Measurement and Classification of Psychiatric Symptoms. London, Cambridge University Press, 1974

Chapter 6

Conclusion

Renee M. Dupont, M.D., Dilip Jeste, M.D.

Psychiatry relies primarily on the observation of behavior for diagnosis; such observations do not necessarily shed light on the underlying disorder. To search for further understanding about the brain through imaging has been seductive, but the interpretation of the results has not been straightforward. In fact, the use of imaging as an approach to answering questions about psychiatric disorders has raised, rather than answered, many questions. For instance, different researchers have produced conflicting results (see Schlegel, Chapter 1, this volume). There are several possible reasons this may be occurring: 1) different patient samples; 2) different control samples; 3) different methods for quantification; and 4) unrecognized contributors to results, such as state-related phenomena. As will be discussed below, such issues must be addressed in future studies if we are to arrive at an understanding of the pathophysiology of affective disorders through imaging.

BRAIN IMAGING RAISES QUESTIONS ABOUT DIAGNOSTIC CATEGORIES

When behavioral or psychiatric dysfunction follows evidence of brain injury, the diagnosis has traditionally been one of an "organic" or "secondary" psychiatric disorder. Patients with such secondary disorders have traditionally been classified as neurologic patients. Those patients without obvious underlying etiologies for behavioral disturbances are, ipso facto, considered psychiatric. Imaging modalities now present new challenges to our nosological schemes and our understanding of disorders. First, structural imaging, such as computed tomography (CT) and magnetic resonance imaging (MRI), has demonstrated in vivo evidence of brain lesions associated with numerous psychiatric disorders, eroding the distinction between primary and secondary disorders. Second, the inconsistency of reports with regard to the presence or absence of definable structural abnormalities has increased rather than decreased the degree of uncertainty regarding etiologies and nosology of symptom clusters in psychiatry. Whether such inconsistencies are methodological or whether they reflect true heterogeneity due to state or diagnostic variance is important. Each new incremental step forward of imaging technology provides advances in resolution and sensitivity for disease discrimination. It is crucial, however, that the new information be incorporated into our diagnostic scheme; clinical information that would allow this must be collected.

ADVANCES

Using CT imaging, Schlegel (Chapter 1, this volume) described subtle changes in the brains of patients with affective disorders. Such alterations in white matter attenuation, also reported by Coffman and Nasrallah (1984, 1985), may be the initial indicators of a disease process involving parenchymal white matter, one that may lead to ventricular enlargement. Furthermore, in a result suggested by this group as well as others, the type of change (e.g., altered attenuation coefficients, focal lesions, global atrophy) may be significantly correlated with clinical subtypes. The limitations of CT (e.g., bone artifact, low resolution in the brain) have shown it to be of limited value despite some pioneering studies demonstrating cortical (Nasrallah et al. 1982), ventricular (Jacoby et al. 1981; Nasrallah et al. 1984; Pearlson et al. 1984, 1985), cerebellar (Lippman et al. 1982), and white matter changes (Coffman and Nasrallah 1984, 1985).

In the elderly, gross structural changes seem to be a clear etiologic factor in the development of affective disorders. Coffey et al. (1988) and Krishnan et al. (1988) reported that there is a high rate of subcortical MRI abnormalities in late-onset affective disorder. Additionally, this group presented some evidence that patients with MRI abnormalities may represent a treatment unresponsive group, requiring electroconvulsive therapy. The most frequent cause of such hyperintense lesions in older individuals is ischemic vascular disease (Awad et al. 1986). It is possible that the primary distinction between those subjects reported by Coffey et al. (1988) and those with poststroke affective disorders studied by Robinson et al. is the degree of neurologic impairment. Thus, MRI has contributed to the blurring of the distinction between primary and secondary affective disorders. Depression, like hemiplegia, may be considered one clinical manifestation of cerebrovascular disease of unknown frequency.

Our center has also reported MRI signal abnormalities in young bipolar patients with no known neurologic illness (Dupont et al. 1990). It remains to be seen whether such lesions are also seen in young unipolar patients. One intriguing question is what process is operating in young patients that would expose them to increased risk for signal hyperintensities and affective disorder.

As outlined by Bryer et al. (Chapter 5, this volume), Starkstein and Robinson have reported that the risk for onset of mania-like symptoms following brain injury is increased by a positive family history for affective illness. The observation of a high rate of structural brain changes in bipolar subjects may be calling our attention to the interplay between genetics and the environment (or experience), which results in the development of affective disorder in predisposed individuals. Thus, the question posed in the chapter by Bryer et al. is increased in complexity from "what lesion leads to affective illness" to "what lesion in the context of what genetic and developmental backgrounds leads to affective illness."

There is some evidence from our work and that of others that those individuals with demonstrable structural abnormalities in the presence of phenotypic display of bipolar illness have a more severe course. Such evidence may indicate that structural changes are part of a distinct phenotype or that different causative factors may contribute to the onset and course of illness. These predisposing factors or events that result in structural changes currently observable on MRI (or as earlier reported with ventricular enlargement or altered attenuation values on CT) may be one of the harbingers of a more severe illness.

It is important that not only destructive processes be studied in the search for underlying structural brain changes in affective disorders. Evidence has been presented for temporal lobe asymmetries in bipolar affective disorder in this volume. Our group has presented preliminary evidence for morphological changes in bipolar disorder involving cortical as well as subcortical structures. Such changes could be the result of either dysgenesis or destruction. Feinberg (1982/83) hypothesized that in some disorders it is anomalous maturation that results in psychiatric disorders: onset in adolescence may be due to age-appropriate neuronal changes that result in the disruption of tenuously maintained equilibrium. Onset in older patients may then be an extended manifestation of this hypothesis when cerebral injury or abnormal aging is the precipitating factor.

The resolution MRI offers provides great advantages in the in vivo study of brain structure; however, disparity between apparently normal anatomy and abnormal function is quite clearly present in some neurologic disorders (e.g., seizure disorder). It is here that functional brain imaging provides clues as to relevant areas of dysfunction in the patient. In Chapter 3 of this volume, by Guze et al., regional abnormalities in cortical and subcortical brain function in bipolar and unipolar disorder are outlined. They have also linked such changes to clinical state. The literature on functional brain imaging in affective disorders is at least as confusing, however, as the literature on the presence or absence of neuropsychological abnormalities associated with these disorders. Perhaps one reason for this lies in the sensitivity of these measurements to state and subtype issues. Only meticulous studies with a longitudinal design will sort this out.

METHODOLOGICAL LIMITATIONS

The ultimate research goal of brain imaging in psychiatric disorders is to understand the relationship between disorders of behavior and hitherto unobservable changes in structure. Beyond this, each imaging technique brings with it promises and limitations. Although MRI offers the chance to localize structural abnormalities, its greatest limitation arises from the fact that molecular perturbations may not result in gross structural changes. Similarly, the limitation of positron-emission tomography (PET) and cerebral blood flow imaging arises from the fact that regional dysfunction may be associated with a state, and not be causative of the affective disorder. Furthermore, regional dysfunction may be the result of distal pathology in much the same way that pervasive brain metabolic changes associated with sleep may be initiated by altered activity within the reticular activating system. PET and cerebral blood flow technologies offer us the chance to localize brain dysfunction associated with poor performance on a specific task and may help us test hypotheses about brain regions involved in the performance of such tasks.

With its capacity for continuous monitoring or mapping of evoked responses, electroencephalography has given us the chance to observe brain function from two extremes of the spectrum. The disadvantage, of course, is our limited ability to localize (resolve) sources of electrical activity. Analogous to PET mapping of cerebral blood flow or metabolism, brain electrical activity mapping may be considered a fingerprint of neuronal activity. Magnetoencephalography, reflecting local flux in magnetic fields, may greatly improve our ability to localize neuronal activity compared with electroencephalography.

CONCLUSION

The real question, whether these technologies will help us understand or diagnose psychiatric disorders, has yet to be answered. In most cases, brain imaging has raised the not too surprising specter of more heterogeneity in psychiatric disorders than we had predicted. Each new technique, each advance in resolution, has partially lifted the curtain, only to reveal even more mystery. The field now must take the time to perform careful prospective studies in psychiatric disorders. In the future, we should be willing to reconsider our nosological biases based on information that new imaging technologies will give us about brain structure and function.

Collaborative studies should be undertaken in an effort to collect information systematically in large numbers of subjects. Such a collaborative effort would permit better interpretation and perhaps better explanation of deviant results, as well as a comparison of disorders for the evaluation of the specificity of findings. It should minimize the variability in results due to sampling error in studies in which the expense of the procedure makes large sample numbers impossible. Correlative, hypothesis-driven studies must be carried out to determine the relationship between structural and functional brain measures in affective disorders. Finally, a major effort must be made to conduct prospective longitudinal studies that can begin to answer questions about the severity of course, development, and possible progression of structural or functional changes, with postmortem validation including gross, microscopic, and molecular assessment. This will require close interaction among the clinician, the radiologist, and the computer programmer.

REFERENCES

Awad IA, Spetzler RF, Hodak JA, et al: Incidental subcortical lesions identified on magnetic resonance imaging in the elderly, I: correlation with age and cerebrovascular risk factors. Stroke 17:1084–1089, 1986

Coffey CE, Figiel GS, Djang WT, et al: Leukoencephalopathy in elderly depressed patients referred for ECT. Biol Psychiatry 24:143–161, 1988

Coffman JA, Nasrallah HA: Brain density patterns in schizophrenia and mania. J Affective Disord 6:307–315, 1984

Coffman JA, Nasrallah HA: Relationships between brain density, cortical atrophy and ventriculomegaly in schizophrenia and mania. Acta Psychiatr Scand 72:126–132, 1985

Dupont RM, Jernigan TL, Butters N, et al: Subcortical abnormalities detected in bipolar affective disorder using magnetic resonance imaging. Arch Gen Psychiatry 47:55–59, 1990

Feinberg I: Schizophrenia: caused by a fault in programmed synaptic elimination during adolescence? J Psychiatr Res 17:319–334, 1982/83

Jacoby RF, Levy R, Bird JM: Computed tomography and the outcome of affective disorder: a follow-up study of elderly patients. Br J Psychiatry 139:288–292, 1981

Krishnan KRR, Goli B, Ellinwood EH, et al: Leukoencephalopathy in patients diagnosed as major depressive. Biol Psychiatry 23:519–522, 1988

Lippman S, Manshadi M, Baldwin H, et al: Cerebellar vermis dimensions on computerized tomographic scan of schizophrenic and bipolar patients. Am J Psychiatry 139:667–668, 1982

Nasrallah HA, McCalley-Whitters M, Jacoby CG: Cortical atrophy in schizophrenia and mania. J Clin Psychiatry 43:439–441, 1982

Nasrallah HA, McCalley-Whitters M, Pfohl B: Clinical significance of large cerebral ventricles in manic males. Psychiatry Res 13:151–156, 1984

Pearlson GD, Garbacz DJ, Breakey WR, et al: Lateral ventricular enlargement associated with persistent unemployment and negative symptoms in both schizophrenia and bipolar disorder. Psychiatry Res 12:1–9, 1984

Pearlson GD, Garbacz DJ, Moberg PJ, et al: Symptomatic, familial, perinatal and social correlates of computerized axial tomography changes in schizophrenics and bipolars. J Nerv Ment Dis 173:42–50, 1985